Real Is the New Natural

Silence the noise blocking *You* from healthy living

By Julie D. Andrews

This book is intended as a reference volume only, not as a medical manual. If you know or suspect that you have a health problem, you should consult a health professional. The author and publisher specifically disclaim any liability, loss, or risk, personal or otherwise, that is incurred as a consequence, directly or indirectly, of the use and application of any of the contents of this book.

ISBN 9781497377165

Cover Design by Simon Avery

Mention of specific companies, organizations, or authorities in this book does not imply endorsement by the author or the publisher, nor does mention of specific companies, organizations, or authorities imply that they endorse this book, its author or the publisher.

First Edition: January 2014

To contact the author regarding speaking engagements and panel participation, please email julie.d.andrews@gmail.com.

For ***my insightful parents****, who told me I was bound to be a writer when I was in 7th grade, curled up in bed, plowing through yet another book (though it'd take me years to fully embrace this path).*

For ***my piano teacher of nearly a decade, Karen Maison****. Ultimately, I couldn't dedicate hours daily to études, but I do apply hours daily to writing (P.S. often while listening to Bach, Chopin and Mozart).*

For yoga, a practice that cracked my heart wide open.

For my late grandfather, ***Nelson David Wirts****, whose tennis-playing, Senior-Olympics-swimming and nightly stretching well into his 70s, along with his inextinguishable spirit, defined healthy living.*

And ***for every person who craves healthier, happier living.*** *You can, and you will, get there.*

Start where you're at.

Start today.

Preface

It just didn't make sense. That's how this book started: utter befuddlement. I had been writing about health, and researching health-related topics and reporting on health news and trends for nearly 10 years, ever since starting out my journalistic career at *Prevention* magazine. All the research I read, and expert sources with whom I spoke, made it clear that healthy lifestyle boiled down to about three simple steps: (1) Eat healthy; (2) Exercise regularly; and, (3) Perform stress reduction daily. And, yet.

And, yet, obesity and diabetes epidemics continued to plague the nation; and, heart disease remained the leading cause of death in the U.S. The fact that all three conditions are preventable just blew my mind. Where was the disconnect? What was the mix-up, hang-up or roadblock? I longed to explore these deeper issues and gain an understanding of the psychology, and the cultural messaging, influencing Americans stuck in trying-but-can't-get-healthy mode. I wanted to observe real people's actions while listening to their comments, challenges and struggles.

Before long, I was on a path jutting away from those easy-to-follow (but somehow rarely followed) healthy-grilling and marathon-training tips-filled articles and getting closer to unraveling what was really going on with people who wanted to be healthy but couldn't quite get there. Watching our culture as purely an observer for six months provided the missing insight and answers. Soon, big, and often unsuspected, barriers began to emerge. Week after week, new pieces of the puzzle surfaced.

One day, obesity was declared a disease (affecting how "obesity treatments" will be covered by insurance), the next I'd stock up on seemingly wholesome yogurts (on sale) only to read labels more closely and feel duped by a not-so-healthy ingredient.

One week, I'd get offered an editing gig where I was never to mention the words "packaged foods," forcing me to ponder whether knowing omission was unethical, the next I'd get disgusted hearing about yet another new fad diet, or being bombarded with crash-diet press releases and assignments (Lose X Pounds in Just Y Weeks Doing Z) signaling bathing-suit season was nearing.

A girl toting a security-blanket jug of pale yellow water would tell me at a Brooklyn BBQ she was on Day 10 of the cleanse Beyoncé did. I'd see the post-baby-bod craze go viral, involving celebs more interested in showcasing their bodies were "back" than coddling their newborns.

And there were labels, and the words on labels, that seemed wholesome and healthy, and yet were plastered on foods that actually were not. There were even those who consistently overdid the good thing known as exercise, to a compulsive degree, pushing their bodies to perform hours of workouts a day while taking in hugely insubstantial amounts of calories, nearly dying by obsession.

With each new message transmitted to me, I'd go to my arsenal of trusted nutrition experts and psychology experts and food-industry and food-science experts and ask them my questions...but *why* do people say, "You look great...have you lost weight?"; and, *how* are we supposed to know what our actual healthy weight should be; and, is juicing *really* healthy; and is the waist on that cover *humanly possible;* and how many calories should a breastfeeding woman *actually* consume; and how long should it *really take* her to safely slim down post-baby; and, what does the vague word on this food label *really* mean; and, *how much* exercise is too much. With those answers, the clutter vanished. What remained? What was really health, what was really happy, what was really safe and what was really smart.

Along with pointing out and dissecting the destructive messaging and obsessive cultural norms coming at us day to day, I decided to also include a few of those "service-y" articles I mentioned earlier with actual tips on what easy methods and systems you can put in place to make healthy living a reality (answering challenges such as: how to keep healthy produce stocked, how to cook healthy at home when there's no time, and what you need to know about food co-ops before joining one, as well as food-label tricks to watch out for and sneaky food-marketing words that should *always* raise an eyebrow). On the more upbeat side, I included uplifting cool, new technologies and startup companies that are finally, at last, making healthy lifestyle easier than ever to achieve.

Put together, it's clear to me now, as it will be to you, how screwy our relationship, as Americans, is to our food, our bodies, our health, and thus, how detached we are from our own paths to happiness, purpose and fulfillment.

Once you start to see the mixed-up, contradictory, confusing and destructive messages constantly bombarding us under the guise of "healthy," you can start to spot them (and disregard them) immediately for what they are: Detractors from simple truths (or the three steps I mentioned earlier: eat healthy; exercise; and, reduce stress). Real is the new natural.

Read on and prepare to disarm the faulty messaging in your path; or, as I like to say, silence the noise blocking *You* from healthy living.

Table of Contents

1. **Why Diets Are the Devil**
Despising the word diet for its false promise. Americans' obsession with weight is harder and harder to escape, yet no less insanity-driving for those promoting healthy lifestyle.

2. **Obesity Is Now Officially A Disease**
So much for America, home of the free, the brave, healthy and youthful. We're now a bunch of sickly, unhappy, immobile and vastly overweight folks.

3. **Why Kim Kardashian's Post-Baby-Bod Magazine Cover Is Damaging to Women**
A tabloid cover brandishing Kim Kardashian's "post-baby" bod…at 40 days…is destructive and insulting to real, everyday women. Plus, three expert nutritionists explain why rapid weight loss is harmful, especially for breastfeeding new moms.

4. **Gwyneth Paltrow Speaks Up about Cleansing's Downsides**
What a breath of fresh air. Gwyneth Paltrow came clean on the wacky side effects, including hallucinations, she experienced doing cleanses in her 20s.

5. **Exploring the Blurring Line Between Ads and Content**
The ever-blurring line between advertisement and content presents shady, new propositions in an ever-changing media landscape and makes us ask—is knowing omission (of, say, the words "packaged foods," ethically wrong?

6. **Duped (Again) by Food Packaging**
Think yogurt is, by nature, a healthy choice? Think again.

7. **Naked Juice Coughs Up $9 Million, Removes "All Natural" from Label**

What the word "natural" on food labels really means. A whole lotta nada.

8. **Food Label Tricks, Not Just for Kids**
Green calorie counts falsely perceived as healthier.

9. **4 Tricks to Keeping Fresh Produce Stocked**
Staying healthy is all about setting up methods and systems.

10. **Christina Applegate Endorses FruitWater, Which Contains No Real Fruit**
Christina Applegate is the buoyant, new poster gal for Coca-Cola's FruitWater, which contains no real fruit or fruit juice. A look into this and other celeb endorsements of junk food.

11. **The Pros and Cons of Joining CSAs**
Which are kind-of like food co-ops. Community Supported Agriculture gets you boxes of fresh produce, all season long. What the joiners are saying.

12. **What Exactly Are Natural Flavors?**
Not nearly as innocent as they sound.

13. **Lady Gaga's Waist on Glamour Cover Is Not Humanly Possible**

Lady Gaga's too-thin waist on her *Glamour* magazine cover is highly disturbing. It sends a dangerous wrong (and unhealthy) message to readers–especially young girls who are at risk for developing eating disorders.

14. **Real Salad! Fresh Salad! In A Vending Machine!**

It's happened and may soon be coming to a shopping mall near you.

15. **HelloFresh Makes Anyone A Gourmet Health Chef**

Meal-prep delivery services take the guesswork out of the healthy-eating equation.

16. **A Look at the Phrase, "You Look Great, Have You Lost Weight?"**

Should commenting on a person's weight be off limits?

17. **Exercising to Death**

Compulsive exercisers just can't get enough, dangerously overdoing a good thing.

18. **Where "Members Only" Means 50-Plus Pounds Overweight**

A gym where everybody knows your name, and your struggle.

Why Diets Are the Devil

I despise the word diet for its false promise. Americans' obsession with weight is harder and harder to escape, and yet no less insanity-driving for those promoting healthy lifestyle.

So, recently, I went to a friend's back-terrace Brooklyn barbecue. In that collaborative summertime fashion, it was potluck, meaning guests carted along side dishes to add to the feast, or slabs of meat or vegetarian meat-like food to be grilled.

As options on the serving table grew, eyes lit up–a fresh salsa, a creamy hummus, veggie sticks, chunks of succulent watermelon, bowls of ripe berries, grilled asparagus.

To the tune of *oohs* and *aahs*, each addition was more enticing than the last, and all of it pleasingly healthy. I noticed that one of the gals wasn't noshing. She, instead, was nursing a large, plastic water bottle containing a pale yellow liquid.

When someone else inquired (I try hard not to butt into others' relationship with food at social gatherings), we all learned that this sprightly woman was on day 10 of a cleanse consisting of water, lemon juice and cayenne pepper.

Only that.

When we next heard, "You know, like the one Beyoncé did, before that big movie," it became clear that the objective behind the "cleanse" was indeed to lose weight.

I confess here and now to keeping a close eye on Tiny the entirety of the party, wanting, no needing to make sure she did not pass out. "Be safe," I said, in the gentlest *I-am-trying-to-understand-but-can t* voice I could muster.

More disappointment ensued when, even at an ashram yoga retreat over the weekend, I happened to always end up standing next to the woman in the food line who, as she approached the buffet, loudly blurted, "It's *way* too easy to overeat here."

Each time I heard this, my agitation swelled. My lips pursed, my eyebrows knitted together, my head cocked. However in the world, I wondered, could it be possible to overdo steamed kale, quinoa, black beans, sweet potatoes, beets, fresh tomatoes, carrots, bananas and apples, sunflower seeds and raisins, this array of wholesome no-salt, no-added-sugar vegetarian plates before us?

It irked me that even at this compassion-fostering, soul-enriching place one could still not detach from food issues; one could still not see food simply for what it was: nourishment.

There are variations on weight obsession, but however mild or severe (I'll never forget how disturbing I found a comment stream filled with women, all women, defending the HCG diet, involving injecting a pregnancy hormone or taking it under-tongue, while researching the *Men s Fitness* article I wrote, "Does the HCG Diet Work?") the case, it is increasingly hard to escape. And I find this entrapment people experience terribly unfortunate. The way people comment on weight vexes me. The way that weight makes people feel about themselves troubles me. It has all this power—hugely undeserving.

Summertime should conjure things frivolous and carefree: swimming in the ocean; twirling in light and flowy fabrics; savoring fresh and juicy produce; running barefoot in the grass, or on the sand; tossing Frisbees in the breeze.

And yet, it's the time when those assignments come around, all the renditions on "Summertime: How to Drop Pounds Fast and Look Great in Your Swimsuit." So instead of looking forward to the liberation of warm-weather leisure, one is programmed to dread having to bare more skin, which is beside summer's grand point: relaxation, adventure, amusement.

I've been writing about health and fitness since my first post-grad-school magazine internship some eight years ago. At first, it struck me as odd how health was so inextricably knotted with diet and weight loss.

If you wanted to write about health, you would, at some point, cover weight-loss success stories, and the latest fad diets, or worse, so-called cleanses. Having seen tons of website traffic reports (at household brands as well as startups), I know the power numbers words like "diet" and "weight loss," among the most highly clicked-on headline words, produce; yet, somehow I dread related assignments. I don't want to give into the country's unhealthy obsession in this way, or to further its ever-expanding reach.

What I never understood was the ambition to lose weight in order to achieve a goal of looking thinner, in say, a bathing suit. What I did always get in a very big way was the pursuit of healthy lifestyle in order to feel better, to banish stress and bad energy, to feel clean and to feel strong, to feel agile and active and youthful and free yet purposeful and focused.

To me, pursuing a healthy lifestyle meant a healthy mind and body; and, by extension, healthy spirit and weight would follow naturally. Managing stress and creating a healthy relationship with food seemed to be key. But these topics were not covered in diet articles, which outlined the do's and don'ts, the rules and limitations, the extractions.

Diets Don't Work

A study in the April 2007 *American Psychologist* journal analyzed 31 long-term studies tracking adults following a range of diets anywhere from two to five years and found that while dieters did shed plenty of pounds in the first six months, the majority regained the initial weight, and more, back.

Indeed, a whopping 83 percent of dieters followed two-plus years re-gained more weight than was lost. Researchers concluded that most study participants would have been better off never having "dieted."

Diets don't work. Point blank. If diets worked, we would have no need to come up with new iterations, because the first ones that came about would have covered it. The word diet, while it has multiple definitions, is most used to mean a regimen of eating and drinking sparingly so as to reduce one's weight.

It is temporary, a means to an end. But what is one to do when the end-goal is reached. Stop? Shifting to a healthy lifestyle is permanent. It's replacing unhealthy shopping-list items with healthy staples, forever. Instead of buying salty chips as a snack, buying unsalted, roasted peanuts, and having only those available at snack time.

Crash Diets Are Not Safe

Recently, I was asked to do an article where the ideal formatting would be, in x amount of weeks, or days, lose y number of pounds by doing z. But that was impossible. I couldn't stand the idea of suggesting that crash diets were safe. My expert nutritionist source pointed out that, for most people, safe weight loss is 1 to 2 pounds per week.

Sweat Is Not Optional

Turns out, someone on a lemon-juice-hot-sauce-whatever-other-flavoring water diet has no energy to safely exercise. And it is fitness and nutrition together that equal healthy lifestyle. Healthy eating alone just doesn't cut it.

We, so often, are a culture seeking easy ways out. Slap a band-aid on. Staple it shut. Pop a vitamin. But healthy lifestyle requires making a conscious choice. It's everyday decision-making. A shift in priorities that puts you in control. Perhaps it even requires making new friends who also prefer evening runs or yoga class to happy hour.

I am aware that, at the time of this writing, according to CDC, more than 35 percent of U.S. adults and about 17 percent of kids ages 2 to 19 are obese.

I'm also aware that the average American consumes three servings of fruits and vegetables daily despite the latest dietary-guidelines recommendation of five to 13 servings (or 2.5 to 6.5 cups), depending on caloric intake.

My favorite way of eating (yes, diet, if you must, but there is nothing temporary about it) is the Mediterranean style. A recent *New England Journal of Medicine* study found this heart-healthy eating style to reduce risk of heart attack and stroke by 30 percent.

Going Mediterranean is about choosing a healthier approach to life—not only by eating mostly fish and whole, plant-based foods but also by regularly exercising and enjoying leisurely, social meals, often with a hearty glass of wine. Try it, but please, whatever you do, don't call it a diet.

Obesity Is Now An Official Disease

So much for America, home of the free, the brave, healthy and youthful. We're now a bunch of sickly, unhappy, immobile and vastly overweight folks.

Here's a real doozy: One in three Americans is now considered diseased. On June 18, 2013, the American Medical Association, a large, clout-carrying physicians' group, went against the recommendations of its own Council on Science and Public Health and forged ahead to officially declare obesity a disease.

The statement read, "Today, the AMA adopted a policy that recognizes obesity as a disease requiring a range of medical interventions to advance obesity treatment and prevention."

The 457 delegates, which represented specialty and state medical societies, overruled the council's recommendation about 60 percent to 40 percent in a vote, reported *The New York Times*.

A disease is defined by Merriam-Webster as "a condition of the living animal or plant body or of one of its parts that impairs normal functioning and is typically manifested by distinguishing signs and symptoms: sickness, malady."

While some physicians agree with the decision, others have been vociferous in their disagreement.

Proponents of the label say that because it impairs body function, obesity is a disease.

Others scratch their heads and ask what the distinguishing signs and symptoms are. They also point out that using body mass index (BMI) alone, to define obesity, (BMIs greater than 30 are considered obese), makes for a faulty diagnostic tool.

In response, the council whose research-based recommendations were pretty much ignored, has already produced a report slamming the AMA's move and urging additional research.

Why does it matter? There are no legal implications, but changing the classification will likely affect whether insurers pay for obesity "treatments."

That's a big deal because Americans shell out some $190 billion a year on higher medical costs due to obesity.

Oh, wait, did you hear that? Yes, exactly. Cha-ching. Such classifications have little to do with achieving a healthier American population.

That's because when we are talking about obesity treatment, this refers to counseling, drugs (such as Qsymia or new-to-market Belviq) and surgery.

Bariatric surgery can cost anywhere between $15,000 to $30,000. Many insurers do not cover this or the cost of obesity drugs.

I'd like to think that access to more treatment means more people battling obesity seeking long-term counseling to gently and thoughtfully work through harmful, self-sabotaging issues. That would make me happy.

But my hunch is that underlying-problem-probing therapy is not the most frequently selected treatment option. This leads me to believe that if and when more "treatments" are covered by insurers, Americans will far too easily come to rely on these quick-fix, side-effect-loaded, body-tampering and costly ways of addressing obesity, otherwise known as excess body fat.

"It's not about blame. It's about action," wrote Keith-Thomas Ayoob, ED.D., R.D., director of the Nutrition Clinic at New York-based Albert Einstein College of Medicine, on a school-sponsored blog. "The sooner we accept this, the sooner we can take control of our health and our lives."

Hear, hear.

Oh, but blaming a disease, or other people, or a job is way easier than taking accountability, seeking support and having to undergo the very hard work and commitment required to make a lifelong shift to healthy lifestyle.

And when given the choice, let's be honest, most of us prefer the path of least resistance.

Supporters of the label also posit that the new classification will prevent society from seeing obesity as only a result of overeating and under-exercising.

Maybe. But probably not. Because here's the thing: As described on Medline Plus, "obesity occurs over time when you eat more calories than you use...Factors that might affect your weight include your genetic makeup, overeating, eating high-fat foods and not being physically active."

How is it wrong for the public to view obesity as related to the type of diet one regularly consumes and the amount of exercise one routinely gets?

We can't sugarcoat this. Consumption of sugar is hugely over the top in the U.S.

An article from the Harvard School of Public Health states, "What's increasingly clear from these early [research] findings is that genetic factors identified so far make only a small contribution to obesity risk—and that our genes are not our destiny."

In other words, we can't blame the global swell in obesity rates on genetic makeup, either.

It's not popular and it's not what many people want to hear. Daily stress reduction, regular exercise (the sweat-producing kind) and healthy, nutritious eating (whether through a support program or self-directed) can, for a great many people, reduce body fat.

To be clear, I do not mean to suggest that losing weight through lifestyle adjustments is easy. It is not. It is actually very hard. And it can be very slow. But the rewards go way beyond actual pounds shed.

Being obese increases risk of diabetes, heart disease, stroke, arthritis and some cancers. This is true. It is a risk factor to be taken tremendously seriously.

But what we're not getting at through these big meetings, and these debates in semantics, is why Americans' relationship to what they eat is so out-of-whack; and what, as a society, we can do to get it back on track.

If it smells rotten, don't eat it.

Why Kim Kardashian's Post-Baby-Bod Magazine Cover Is Damaging to Women

A tabloid cover brandishing Kim Kardashian's "post-baby" bod…at 40 days…is damaging and insulting to real, everyday women. Plus, three expert nutritionists explain why rapid weight loss is harmful, especially for breastfeeding new moms.

So there we were, putzing around where Fulton Street meets the East River, otherwise known as the South Street Seaport. (As an aside, we had zoomed down on our bike-share rides; since Citibike launched some 60 days ago, New Yorkers have pedaled 3-million-miles-and-counting: Success!).

Après patronizing the limping-back-to-life-post-Sandy port, my boyfriend and I popped into Duane Reade to buy light bulbs. As we waited in line to pay, *Psst,* the tabloid headline seemed to whisper to me, *"New Mom Kim: How She Lost 50 Lbs in 40 Days."*

"You have got to be kidding me," to my boyfriend I said with a sigh.

But it was not a joke. It was a real magazine, to be picked up and bought; to be rifled through for the details.

So, let's see. Kim Kardashian gave birth to her baby girl with Kanye West, North West, on June 15. Here we were, just 42 days later, and here it was?

Yes, we knew this was coming. But, my God, already?

Now, to be fair, Kim Kardashian is not quoted in this article. This was not an exclusive interview that had been granted to the publication. There are quotes from mysterious, unnamed friends.

The cover reads: *"How She Lost 50 Lbs in 40 Days. Only 1,200 calories a day and grueling three-hour workouts."* At the time of this article, there has been no confirmation that Kim Kardashian actually shed 50 Lbs. in 40 days.

Odd that when the Editorial Director at the site where this essay will first appear went to purchase a photo, he could not locate one on Splash News, Corbis, AP, Getty Images, Reuters, Veer, oh, and did I mention Shutterstock?

Indeed, our sisters over at Jezebel claim that the photo is no post-baby bod at all; but rather, a photo dating back to 2012 that was uploaded by a fan at that time. (Way to research, Ladies!)

So, there are no post-baby photos to be found and it's been reported that Kim Kardashian is allegedly planning to make her big post-baby-bod reveal on her mom, Kris Jenner's, talk show that debuted on July 15, to the throngs of fans champing at the bit to get a glimpse of her body (hey, I don't understand it either).

But whether or not the story is 100 percent true is beside the point I'd like to make here.

Everyday women should be able to pay for their groceries at the register without being bombarded with such body-obsessive ridiculousness.

More important, these you-are-your-body message blasts are more than trifling; they are harmful and irresponsible.

Even if one real-life, post-partum new mom flipped through to find out how Kim *"Got Her Body Back!"* and thought, "Hey, why don't I try some rendition of this get-fit-quick scheme," that's a big problem.

Imagine the woman who does not buy the magazine but just reads the numbers on the cover: 5o lbs in 40 days; 1,200 calories a day; three-hour workouts. (Even when I was marathon training, I never logged three hours of workouts in a day; and if I did, my fuel needs would be drastically higher.)

Unsafe, You Say?

Yes. Let me enumerate the ways.

1. For starters, breastfeeding women need to eat more.

"This is not the right message," says Lisa Young, PhD, RD, a nutritionist and adjunct professor in NYU's Department of Nutrition, Food Studies and Public Health.

"If you are breastfeeding, you should consume more calories not fewer. Eating less could compromise the nutrients going to the baby."

Jennifer McDaniel, LDN, RDN, a registered dietitian nutritionist and Academy of Nutrition and Dietetics Spokeswoman, concurs. "Most experts agree that women need an additional 300 calories a day to support breastfeeding."

La Leche League recommends no dieting at all until a breastfeeding woman is two months post-partum, so she can build an adequate milk supply.

2. Psychological pitfalls of dieting do not bode well for bonding with Baby.

"Losing weight quickly will never be a good thing," says Dr. Young, pointing out the psychological downsides of dieting: "Hunger, irritability, sluggishness and the high probability that all the weight lost will be re-gained."

It's tough to be a coddling, goo-goo-ga-ga-ing cuddle-bug of a new mom when you're fending off hunger pangs.

And here's the thing, adds McDaniel, a mom herself who is pregnant with her second child, "If and when the weight is later regained, it will not likely be muscle but fat. This means that body composition has been compromised."

3. Rapid weight loss is harmful.

Of course it's eyecatching, 50 pounds in 40 days. It's astonishing because it's way beyond what nutritionists suggest.

"Losing weight at that rate could only be done with questionable and most likely unsafe methods that would not be recommended," says McDaniel.

She adds that a healthy, post-partum get-back-to-pre-baby goal would be to drop 1 to 2 pounds of weight per week. Drastic the difference, no?

"Faster weight loss could result in loss of lean body mass (muscle) and skeletal mass, drained energy for Mom and Baby, inadequate breast milk production, decreased immunity, and delayed post-delivery recovery," says McDaniel.

Adds Gina Neill, RD, LDN, a registered dietician, who spent years educating post-partum women on proper mom-and-baby nutrition in obstetrics and neonatal units before founding Glow Nutrition, "It's called 'skinny fat,' and refers to the dry and brittle skin, softer physique, and slower metabolism that shedding pounds rapidly can lead to. That's because it's not only fat that's lost. Things like lean body mass, or muscle, also take a hit."

The average weight gain during pregnancy for a healthy woman (meaning with a BMI between 18.5 and 24.9) is between 25 to 35 pounds, according to the Institute of Medicine 2009 guidelines.

So, let's say a woman gained 35 pounds over her nine-month pregnancy. Now, let's say she lost one pound per week after delivering her baby. It would take 35 weeks to return to her pre-baby weight.

That's nearly nine months. Isn't that nifty how that works out, and how it makes sense. Nine months on; nine months off.

Now, if she lost, let's say, two pounds per week, that would be about four-and-a-half to five months.

Pregnant women can also expect to shed up to 10 pounds during childbirth, says Neill, when the baby, placenta and other tissues leave the body, so even if a woman lost less than a pound per week, she could still potentially return to pre-baby form in nine months.

4. Priorities, people.

"Dieting is deprivation—not the kind of mentality you want to have as a new mom," says McDaniel. "If there's especially a time to have patience with your body, it is just after having a baby. It took nine months to put that weigh on. It is okay and normal if it takes that long to take it off."

Women experience many changes at this time in life. They have new responsibilities. They are trying to care for newborns. Their hormones are shifting. If they choose to breastfeed, they are trying to feed their babies with their own bodies. The primary focus for most women is, as it should be, caring for their newborn and adjusting to life as a new mom.

"I recommend that women take in at least 1,800 calories a day for adequate milk production," says McDaniel.

Neill points out that determining calorie needs should be based on factors including height, weight, age, activity level and whether a woman is breastfeeding.

The focus should be on eating for nourishment, so new moms will have enough energy to care for a newborn and to fuel moderate, regular exercise which can keep her body healthy and mood positive.

This means, adding to her diet, says McDaniel, with fruits and vegetables, lean proteins, healthy fats, calcium-rich dairy. And let's not forget healthy whole grains, adds Neill.

In other words, additional, burdensome pressures to "get her body back" have no place. Because that new baby mama is so much more than her body.

Gwyneth Paltrow's Speaks Up on Cleansing's Downsides

What a breath of fresh air. Gwyneth Paltrow came clean on the wacky side effects, including hallucinations, she experienced doing cleanses in her 20s.

Yes, I used the words fresh air and Gwyneth Paltrow in back-to-back sentences, implying that her reveal was refreshing. Deal with it.

Hate on her if you must (it seems to be a new national pastime) but I applaud her. It is encouraging to see a celebrity speak the truth, openly and honestly, about the hardships she has put her body through in order to look a certain way, that being slim, slender, svelte, you name the hot-bod adjective. All the things her younger, 20-something self did that her seasoned, 40-year-old self now regrets having done.

What She Said

In a column she wrote in *The Daily Telegraph*, a London-based newspaper, on how to create a lean body shape, Paltrow wrote, "I've done juice cleanses in the past, and in my twenties I did Master Cleanse which left me hallucinating after 10 days."

In an online medical dictionary, it reads that "in the final stages of starvation, adult humans experience a variety of neurological and psychiatric symptoms, including hallucinations and convulsions, as well as severe muscle pain and disturbances in heart rhythm."

Well, look at that.

Unfortunately, Paltrow's admission wasn't a shocker to any of us, *n ést-ce pas*? Instead it was a sad reminder of the pressures put on celebs to look a certain way, no matter the cost to their health and well-being.

But when Paltrow proceeded with a warning, it was a step in the much-needed, right-message direction: "Be aware: a juice detox can crash your metabolism and lead to future weight gain."

Why This Is Good News

Holla. If I could ship this out to all the young girls (and boys) considering their first cleanse, or if I could thumb-tack this to their bulletin boards and highlight it in pretty colors, and heart-shaped doodles, you know that I would. Down with the cleanse, detox, fast, juice diet, whatever-you-want-to-call-it.

"There is no scientific evidence to indicate that following any type of cleansing diet provides any health benefits," says Joy Dubost, PhD, RD, an Academy of Nutrition and Dietetics Spokesperson and founder of Dubost Food & Nutrition Solutions.

"Cleanses and detox diets are typically done under the premise that your body cannot rid itself of toxins without needed assistance. This is not the case," says Dr. Dubost. "Your body naturally cleanses itself and has a built-in detox system through the liver, gastrointestinal tract, lungs and kidneys. I would not recommend following a cleansing or detoxing diet."

We've heard about many celebs cleansing. Years back, Beyoncé Knowles admitted on the Oprah show that she lost 20 pounds on a Master Cleanser to slim-down for her *Dreamgirls* role.

Howard Stern's sidekick Robin Quivers relayed to *People* magazine that she shrunk down to 145 from 215 pounds in 2004, when she did the controversial Master Cleanser on three separate occasions.

But rarely do we hear from stars about the grueling realities of what fasting for some 10 days is really like.

How many times have you been at a shindig trying to have a rollicking, good time only to hear about the cleanse Beyoncé did (as if, "Hey, that diva did it so it must be okay"); or worse, seen the jug, that ever present reminder of the struggles women (and sometimes men) face, and lug around with them.

When the downsides are mentioned, such as on blogs, it can seem as if suffering through a cleanse is some sort of a (terribly misplaced) badge of honor. In the name of Thin, I overcame (or just plain ignored) the pain—my body's cry for tender-loving attention and care.

In a well-reported *New York Times* article from years back, nutritionist Joy Bauer once estimated that those on the cleanse who guzzled six, eight-ounce glasses of the lemon juice, cayenne pepper, maple syrup, water concoction daily—six to 12 glasses daily are recommended—consumed only 650 calories. (The Master Cleanse also involves drinking a glass of sea-salt-water mixture in the a.m.; and, herbal laxative tea in the p.m. *Mmmm*, delish!)

"The reality is that any extremely low-calorie plan, such as the Master Cleanse, will cause significant weight loss. Some other juice cleanses/detoxes are even lower in calories. But this is absolutely starving yourself. After just 24 to 48 hours, the body starts to slow down and conserve. The body understands this as starvation," says Marjorie Nolan Cohn, MS, RD, author of *Belly Fat Fix* and an Academy of Nutrition and Dietetics National Spokesperson.

The calorie intake required for a person's optimal health depends on factors such as height, weight, age, activity level and body composition.

"The general rule of thumb in the professional nutrition world is a minimum 1,200 to 1,400 calories for women to maintain a healthy body weight; and, for men, a minimum of 1,400 to 1,600 calories. More often, most people need more calories," says Cohn. (As you'll see online, USDA's estimated calorie intakes based on gender and activity level are substantially higher.)

Additional characteristic symptoms of starvation include diminished sex drive (hello, weak and grumpy vixen); and, more dangerously, shrinkage of the heart, lungs, ovaries; lower body temperature and sensitivity to cold; anemia; irritability; difficulty concentrating.

The list goes on, but I'll stop there. The point is starvation is bad. Very bad. In fact, starvation can lead to death.

Even after all that bulge battling, guess what?

"The weight doesn't stay off," says Cohn. "Because once one starts eating again, the metabolism is compromised and burning fewer calories. The deprivation of all food one endures on a cleanse sets him or her up to want to eat all those foods they've been denying themselves after it's over. Plus, the body is craving calories/sugar to replace glycogen in the muscles. Combine this desire for food with the body's real need to have it, and this is absolutely a set-up for disaster, in the form of binge-eating."

Celeb Mish-Mash

When is the last time you read a celeb cover-story that was truly interesting? Actually showed you a glimpse of who the star was as a person—hurdles, struggles, warts and all?

Nowadays, producing a celebrity cover story involves a heckuva rigamarole. The gate-keeper publicist keeps close tabs on what is published. Often, the publicist approves much of the information that appears in a cover-story before it goes to print.

If something unflattering (read authentic) does make it through the cracks, all hail the wrath. Calls will be made. The relationship between the magazine and the publicist can falter; and, access to the celeb can subsequently be denied, unless the unspoken rules are obeyed.

Another likely scenario: Even when access is granted; interviews can take the form of piddly, 20-minute phone calls. A friend of mine recently filled me in that she was charged with writing a thousand-words-long cover story having been granted 20 minutes of phone-time with the celeb (*pssst*, a big reason why professional writers should consider investing in LexisNexis research accounts). Even if celebs want to get real with it, it can be hard for them to get their message out if it differs from the message others want them to give.

The History of Cleansing

Everybody has heard of the the Master Cleanse (also called the lemonade diet), which is the brain child of Stanley Burroughs. It dates back to the 1940s, when he first presented it as a way to treat ulcers and other internal maladies. The natural-health enthusiast then published it as a book in the 70s, and The Master Cleanser, was an overnight success. Initially, people who were already rather healthy looked at it as a way to banish impurities and toxins (think additives and insecticides) from their bodies. It's still a money-making franchise that offers books and master-cleanse kits for sale. It has been touted in magazines and on websites as recently as 2012.

Young Girls Dream (Not So) Big

Why does it matter? People are curious about celebs. They read about celebs; they mirror celebs' actions. They even listen to celebs' advice more closely than that of practicing nutritionists, dieticians and doctors.

And get this: Celebrity magazines sell more copies than the total sales of magazines in the food, games, health, automotive, home, lifestyle and teen categories combined, according to a presentation by Gil Brechtel, president and CEO of the Magazine Information Network (MagNet), at the MPA/PBAA Retail Marketplace conference in June 2013.

A friend of mine who works at a magazine where the reader demographic is young women in their teens and 20s recently told me that when asked about their career aspirations and hopes for the future, the vast majority of responses from the young, female readers expressed a desire for fame.

Only that. Being famous. These are the reasons why Gwyneth Paltrow's warning against cleansing was a good deed. Pure and simple. (Now, her admission to smoking on Saturdays? Not so good. But, hey, at least it was honest.)

Key Takeaway

"If you want to fast and cleanse," says Dr. Dubost, "I would suggest drinking more water, increasing the amount of fiber in your diet and incorporating probiotics into the diet."

A good dietary approach, and one that will not negatively affect your metabolism, is to follow a life-long eating pattern of healthy eating, meaning fruits and vegetables, whole grains, low-fat dairy and lean protein.

Eliminating any of these food groups, says Dr. Dubost, can potentially set you up for a deficiency of essential nutrients.

"Master Cleanse and other such products and plans can be dangerous because they eliminate essential nutrients. One can feel weak, irritable, constipated and lack energy."

And then there are those hallucination spells. Damn it.

Exploring the Blurring Line Between Ads and Content

The ever-blurring line between advertisement and content presents shady, new propositions in an ever-changing media landscape and raises the question—is knowing omission of health information ethically wrong?

Recently, a gal I met years back in an NYU editing course, with whom I'd grab the occasional Eataly glass of Malbec, emailed to tell me she'd heard of an interesting opportunity and put forth my name.

In my line of work, it's always a lovely, unexpected gift to have a friend who knows you, your passions and your work, think of you and recommend you when not-widely-advertised gigs crop up.

Heaps of editorial projects never bubble up to the general job-board surface; if and when they do, it's often a formality…due diligence…after the top candidates have already been identified.

What happens first? Knowledge of the gig gets disseminated through an intricate web of "Who do you know?" calls, emails and inquisitions.

At the time of this posting, all the assigns, projects and clients in my work pie landed in my lap either directly from a friend, or from a friend-of-a-friend who kindly made a referral.

When the aforementioned pal said this gig involved health and wellness idea-pumping and writing and editing a batch of monthly content—on a remote-basis, the *only* way I roll these days—my ears perked.

Within days, I received the anticipated reach-out via email and an info-gathering chat was arranged post haste.

The first 15 minutes of the call were standard fare. Talk revolved around editing styles, idea generation, contacts and sources, health reporting and coverage and strategies for selecting and managing a team of writers.

Then, the conversation veered off-course.

There's one other thing we need to discuss, the person on the other end of the call said to me, tapering off to a mysterious pause.

"Do you have anything…out there…railing against processed foods?"

Hm. This seems fishy, I thought.

Though I would not call it railing, merely service-y and informative, most every nutritionist with whom I have spoken through the years—and I talk with quite a few on a regular basis—at some point has mentioned the importance of consuming more fruits and vegetables, the whole, raw sort, and less processed junk parading as food (you know, the items lining the food stores' inner aisles).

What's more, both of the ebooks I ghostwrote stressed the importance of severely limiting, if not entirely cutting, processed junk from one's diet and getting back to fresh-produce basics.

The hiring manager went on to explain that the site being built was "sponsored." It would be sponsored by a large, household-recognized company that made and sold processed foods.

She was unable to tell me the company's name—the two parties were in final talks that would conclude in three weeks' time. The content generated was to be health-focused, service-y, chock full of nutritionist- and doctor-recommended healthy-lifestyle advice.

But, here's the kicker: There was to be strictly no mention whatsoever of processed foods on the site.

Is Omission Wrong?

At first it was laughable to me. However could you discuss health—look the (preventable) health epidemics plaguing the nation in the eye (at press time, obesity affects more than one-third of adults in the U.S.; diabetes affects nearly 26 million Americans ages 20-plus; one in three Americans has high blood pressure; and, heart disease remains the number one killer of adults in the U.S.)—and fail to mention processed foods?

Some 70 percent of the nations' calories come from processed foods.

Pulitzer Prize-winning *New York Times* reporter Michael Moss, in his new best-selling book, *Salt Sugar Fat: How the Food Giants Hooked Us*, details America's unregulated food-industry giants' use of unhealthy methods to get consumers addicted to their brands and products.

A *New York Times* article reports that "Americans eat 31 percent more packaged food than fresh food," and that "A sizable part of the American diet is ready-to-eat meals, such as frozen dinners and pizzas, and salty and sweet snacks."

The problem is not processed foods, per se, but the ingredients most tend to contain, and often in excessive amounts (such as the aforementioned fat, sodium and sugar).

For example, looking just at salt, the American Heart Association reports that up to 75 percent of the sodium in the average American diet is from salt added to processed and restaurant foods.

Alas, no chuckles poured into the phone lines as I was asked again and again my thoughts on processed foods—and whether I would be able to refrain from covering them as a topic on this health site, were I charged with its content creation and management.

Scanning years of clips in my brain quickly, I knew scads of my articles trumpeted the importance of real, whole foods and advised the near-banning of powders, boxes, cans and bags of junk.

They included information on how to scan the needlessly complicated food labels on processed foods.

Indeed, turns out I have been quite vocal also about my support of the Mediterranean style of eating, where the emphasis is placed on, you guessed it, real foods (think fruits, vegetables, nuts, seeds and fish) and sweets and red meat are avoided.

Later, we went on to discuss the monthly rate for the work, which luckily, was also laughable. (As your own agent, your own boss, your own "decision-maker at large," the one thing you absolutely need to know is your value; and the one thing you must own is your rate. Because at a certain point, you will have produced, edited, proofread, analyzed, tracked, written so much content that your gut will be well trained, your eye sharp, your ability to compete healthy, your source book fat and your speed ultra-fast, all of which your rate should reflect.)

But, I digress. What I wondered next, while the woman kept talking, and I stopped listening, was whether health content could be guilty by omission.

If one wrote about every health topic under the sun (there are so many) and offered valuable advice—but failed to mention one topic, arguably one of the biggest culprits of America's ballooning girth and related decline in health, would this be wrong?

Being Held Accountable

For me, I knew the answer was yes, it would be wrong. Knowing omission was not something to which I could agree.

Leaving out the guilty parties—not holding them accountable for deceptive advertising, for the ridiculously over-the-top amounts of fat, sugar and sodium in our foods, and long lists of ingredients consumers just like me can't pronounce let alone translate—because Big Food was sponsoring the site?

Oh, Hell no. Wasn't going to happen. Readers deserve more than that. The public deserves not to be talked down, or dumbed down, to anymore.

A person trying to shop smarter and eat healthier shouldn't have to carry flashcards in his or her wallet to be able to recognize all the secret code names added sugar goes by on food labels (a Harvard School of Public Health article lists 23).

A right and a wrong don't make a right. And in this business, if you don't have conviction, good luck to you. If you don't sincerely want the answers, if you don't want to understand better why troubling things are the way they are, if you do not authentically believe in what you are reporting and writing and presenting to the public, then yes, you are a fraud.

I never sent my resume the next day. Someone else surely did. Because a writer needs to eat; and to a certain group, writing is like breathing, it is life-sustaining.

Ultimately, a sponsored site run by an advertiser is different than a site run by a publisher, the same way an advertorial is different than an article.

Some things can't be bought. Some things are all you have. Your name. People's trust in your drive and search for truth and understanding. Your integrity.

At some point, every health, wellness and fitness writer has read enough research to know what is right, and what is wrong, what methods have proven to actually help people get on a healthy track and what methods do not work. Each will have to decide to be part of the problem, or to try to be part of the solution. Me, I want to be part of the solution.

Also, I must admit, I don't like it when people try to tell me what *not* to write about.

Duped (Again) by Food Packaging

Think yogurt is, by nature, a healthy choice? Think again.

Low-fat! Probiotic Formula! Vitamins A & D Added! Supports Immunity and Digestive Health!

And, by the way, if you read that small-print list tucked away in the ingredients section on this here La Yogurt, you will also find High Fructose Corn Syrup (yep, no colorful banner or burst to amplify that during your split-second buying decision).

It happened again. Yep, I was in a mad rush, just like you likely often are when you realize you are hungry and end up buying food.

I had popped into a convenience store for a notebook, of all things, and as I made a beeline for the register (I mean the you-don't-need-to-interact-with-a-human-soul-ever-again self checkout), there in a refrigerated display case I spotted 89-cent yogurts.

I mean, by nature, all yogurt is healthy, right? I'm buying yogurt. I'm eating healthfully. I'm feeling good.

Wrong.

This, I knew. But, oh, such a good price, I thought (because, let's be honest, with the ever-rising cost of foods, we're eyeballing cost, in addition to the is-this-food-or-junk checklist).

I crammed my arms with as many yogurts as they'd hold, along with my spiral, and punched a hole in my purse, where I'd soon dump the lot.

Now, I *checked* the added sugars amount listed. And, I *checked* the sodium, and the saturated fat. And, of course, I scouted the calcium percentage.

But, you see, I failed to check the ingredients list with that magnifying glass now requisite when purchasing any item under the processed-food umbrella (which, yep, includes yogurts posturing as wholesome and innocent, too).

Hey, I was in a hurry. I forgot the is-this-food checklist. And I had been recently miffed at my favorite probiotics yogurt brand, Stonyfield, when I realized recently that one serving of a certain flavor contained 35 g of sugars.

(Why is this problematic, you ask? I don't know about you, but I don't precisely measure out my one cup of yogurt. I reach for the container and spoon it out until the bowl looks full. Also, keeping in mind that different groups recommend different daily sugar limits, ensuring consumers' persistent befuddlement, American Heart Association recently released sugar guidelines that recommend adult women limit added-sugars intake to about 5 or 6 teaspoons (20 to 25 grams) daily; men, 9 teaspoons (36 grams daily.)

Translation? One sweet, little yogurt and you're sugar-maxed for the day. (Did I mention the average American sucks down more than 22 teaspoons of added sugars daily?)

Right, so this Low-fat! Probiotic Formula! Vitamins A & D Added! yogurt was good. Or at least seemingly better. This

Supports Immunity and Digestive Health yogurt contained 26 g of sugar (hey, less than 35, but, who knew, still more than I should have over the course of one day. Now, if only the FDA would only require brands tell us how much of listed sugars were naturally occurring, such as in fruit, and how much were added, such as HFCS.)

Still, I looked forward to eating those yogurts.

Got home. Loaded those babies into the fridge with that sense of taking care of my body and having bought something health-promoting. I grabbed one to eat right away. I was hungry! It was yogurt! Having just a moment more than I did whirlwinding 'round the store, I glanced the ingredients label…just because.

There were those pesky, food-politics-ridden words: High fructose corn syrup, ingredient number three listed, after sugar.

Duped again. Now when I say duped by a food label, I mean that I *did* glance at the packaging before purchasing, but quickly, and at one thing (such as the sugar amount) but not at another (such as the ingredient list). I spent my hard-earned dollars on the product and realized, just as I went to dig my utensil in and enjoy, that I was about to shovel in a big, nasty ingredient.

I ate that damn yogurt. Quickly. I was hungry. Then I threw the rest away, feeling hugely defeated.

This has happened to me several other times recently, which, of course, was the impetus for this column. Watch your labels, Dear Readers:

What it was: Stonyfield Yogurt, a brand that I like heaps. It has organic ingredients and probiotics and does offer a whopping 35% bone-fortifying calcium per serving.

Why it's a dupe: Some flavors, such as strawberry, also contain, I discovered, 35 g of sugars per serving (remember, as it stands on nutrition labels right now, there's no way to tell how much of "sugars" is added and how much is natural, for example, from within fruit). Why this much sugar? I don't want it. I'd still buy your product without it. Really.

What it was: A Blue Bunny FrozFruit Fat-Free All Natural Flavor Made With Real Fruit Chunky Pineapple Frozen Fruit Bar

Why it's a dupe: Got home, unwrapped, and discovered, under a package flap, this seemingly simple treat also contained, yep, high fructose corn syrup, followed by corn syrup. Boo.

What it was: Gummy vitamins, the Nature Made Adult Gummies Multi, also admittedly purchased in a mad rush.

Why it's a dupe: Yep, you got it, corn syrup, listed as ingredient number one (remember, ingredients are listed by weight).

What it was: Black Beans, Trader Joe's

Why it's a dupe: Don't get me wrong. I love Trader Joe's. It is my number one, top-pick food store. But while I looked at the amount of sodium per serving on this can, which was 440 mg, I failed to notice on my hasty label glance that one can contained three servings. And, well, you know me, I like to save time, and will often have a can (yes, the whole can) of black beans (Folate! Fiber! Protein! Iron! Oh, right, we don't see such banners on boring, healthy-food packaging) with garlic, onions and melted, shredded low-fat cheese for lunch. So that lunch would contain 1,320 mg of sodium. While the American Heart Association recommends limiting sodium to 1,500 mg daily, the average American consumes a whopping 3,400 mg daily. (Funny that when I looked online for the labels, often the ingredients lists and/or number of servings per package were not included, all of which you need to truly assess a food product's health value.)

Key Takeaway: Purchasing healthful food nowadays, especially on a budget, requires a serious amount of knowledge; but what's scary, is that even when you have a basic know-how, you likely don't have the time to dedicate to the science of considering all aspects of a food product's label before committing to a purchase. No one has this kind of time. No one I know, at least. And the companies that make processed foods very much know this. They know we see those Probiotics! Vitamins A & D! Low-fat! bursts and we grab.

So what's one to do? Well, remember: You want something done right? Do it yourself. Make your own frickin' fruit pops.

We did. Last night. Using a blender purchased from Duane Reed (patience, not our strongest virtue), our $2 Ikea plastic pop molds, fresh mint, watermelon, cucumber and a dollop of honey. Total time spent, including buying produce and blender: 40 minutes. For reals.

We just tested them and guess what? They taste better. Way better. My man and I even served them to guests last night. They're the real deal. Go whole, go fresh, go no-gimmicks, do-it-yourself. You *do* have time for this. Trust me.

Naked Juice Coughs Up $9 Million, Removes "All Natural from Label

What the word "natural" on food labels really means. A whole lotta nada.

Ah, a burst of good news for the trying-to-be-healthy, tired-of-being-lied-to consumer. Isn't that encouraging. In a $9 million settlement reached in July, Naked Juice's parent company, PepsiCo, agreed to refund consumers who bought certain Naked Juice products and decided to remove the words "All Natural" from the juice's packaging.

On August 27, a settlement website, NakedJuiceClass.com, sprouted up, where consumers can request refunds.

The class action lawsuit, filed in a district court of California, was consolidated from five class action complaints filed against Naked Juice (owned by PepsiCo).

The plaintiffs alleged that Naked Juice (you know, that $4/bottle oh-so-pure-seeming juice) made false health claims on the brand's packaging, namely that it used the marketing words "All Natural" on its bottles, allegedly intending to lure consumers the company knew would pay more for seemingly authentic, wholesome, naturally healthy juice.

In addition to the words "All Natural," the brand's use of the following terms on its juice bottles was also brought under scrutiny:

*** All Natural Fruit**

*** All Natural Fruit + Boosts**

*** 100% Fruit**

*** 100% Juice**

*** Non-GMO**

*** From Concentrate**

PepsiCo refuted the claims. The company stands by its Naked Juice products. However, it has also decided to no longer use the words "All Natural" on the juice packaging.

The beverage company will refund consumers who purchased certain of its juice products between September 27, 2007 and August 19, 2013. (File a claim and find a list of eligible products online.)

The refund here, up to $75 for those with proof of purchase and up to $45 for those without, is only half of this win.

The big score here are the holes poked in such enticing, deceptive "health" marketing terms plastered on labels, such as "All Natural."

It's a way to water down these words in the consumers' minds and remind buyers that rather than trusting a product to *tell them* it is healthy, it is far better to check labels and stick with the truly all-natural (as in from the earth) foods such as raw, real and whole produce.

The lawsuit claimed that Naked Juice/PepsiCo violated consumer protection statutes as well as federal and state laws regarding advertising, labeling and marketing of some of its products since they contained ingredients such as genetically modified soy.

A statement detailing the settlement of the class action lawsuit read: "The lawsuit claims that the [Naked Juice Products] contain ingredients that are not 'All Natural' and contain GMOs, or Genetically Modified Oganisms."

On Naked Juice's Facebook page, which has amassed some 785,357 followers, the company states in its About Us section, "In 1983, on the beach in Santa Monica, California, a line was drawn in the sand, metaphorically speaking. A line between real and fake, between truth and falsehood, between juice and the previous lack thereof."

Oh, goodness, that seems rather hilarious at the present time, no?

Another descriptive blurb on the social media page reads, "This is fruit's higher purpose. Only the best ingredients go into our bottles. Just the healthiest fruits and vegetables, and a heaping handful of yum." Well that and allegedly some synthetic ingredients and GMOs.

To be fair, it shouldn't just be brands like PepsiCo's Naked Juice and Kellogg's Kashi (who faced a similar lawsuit) that are under the gun here.

The public needs to hold agencies such as the FDA and the FTC, those charged with regulating product advertising, accountable.

That's because, as Marion Nestle, PhD, MPH, the Paulette Goddard Professor of Nutrition, Food Studies, and Public Health at New York University, pointed out on her Food Politics blog back in March, 2012, "The meaning of 'natural' . . . many people perceive as the equivalent to organic or healthy. As I've said before, it isn't. Natural has no regulatory meaning."

Got that? Remember it. Don't be bamboozled.

The FDA does not have a definition for natural and does not offer regulatory guidance on its usage. Nor does the FTC.

Dr. Nestle goes on to explain that research shows that shoppers associate the word "natural" with the words "healthy" or "minimally processed" foods—even though the word "natural" is actually meaningless on a label.

The managers of the brand's Facebook page must have been working overtime to handle all the comments left from disappointed consumers (who says activism is dead?).

Some consumers' comments claimed that some of their other comments had been deleted; some consumers' comments, such as a from a gal named Shannon, were answered in the comments section:

Naked Juice: "Hi Shannon, hope this helps. Naked juice and smoothies will continue to be labeled "non-GMO," and until there is more detailed regulatory guidance around the word "natural"—we've chosen not to use "All Natural" on our packaging. To ensure that our consumers most concerned about that issue can feel even more confident about Naked products, we plan to enlist an independent, third-party to confirm our non-GMO status across the entire Naked brand portfolio. From our ingredients to our practices, we always strive to do the right things."

One of the attorneys who filed a PepsiCo lawsuit (in September 2011) on behalf of a Texas resident, Yvette Golan, also filed a suit against Kashi's parent company, Kellogg's.

Despite the biggie parent companies lawyering up, neither case was dismissed. Golan has said that she plans to file cases in Florida, New Jersey, New York and Hawaii in the future.

Since back in 2012, there has been an spike in lawsuits filed by plaintiffs alleging companies falsely advertised products as "all natural" or "100% natural" when the products contained synthetic ingredients or genetically modified organisms, reports LegalNews.com, which lists past defendants, including Ben & Jerry's, Frito-Lay, Snapple and Trader Joe's among other household brands.

Remember, Dear Reader, "All Natural": don't believe the type. You're way smarter than that.

Food Label Tricks, Not Just for Kids

Green calorie counts falsely perceived as healthier.

Add this to the litany of label tricks to avoid. In addition to checking amount per serving, number of servings and ingredient lists, now keep an eye out for label color, which can be as deceiving as meaningless words like "All Natural" in holding sway over buyers' decisions.

In a recent Cornell University study, participants perceived a candy bar with a green calorie count as more health-promoting than a candy bar with a red calorie count—even when the number of calories was exactly the same.

So, in effect, poor-nutrition food products with such green labels—for example, Snickers bars and M&M's—can play tricks on consumers' minds.

Turns out seeing green, a color that research has found may boost creativity, whose shades symbolize growth and nature, can actually boost the perceived healthfulness of foods, but here's the bizarre part—this holds true especially among consumers who "place high importance on healthy eating," according to an article in the *Cornell Chronicle.*

It's increasingly common to spot eye-catching calorie labels on the front of food packaging now, including on candy-bar wrappers.

And currently, "There's little oversight of these labels," said study researcher Jonathon Schuldt, an assistant professor of communications who is also director of Cornell's Social Cognition and Communication Lab.

"Our research suggests that the color of calorie labels may have an effect on whether people perceive the food as healthy, over and above the actual nutritional information conveyed by the label, such as calorie count," said Schuldt.

When he had students imagine feeling hungry, then showed them candy bars with green or red calorie labels, they perceived the green-label bars as healthier. But the calorie counts were identical.

A repeated experiment with online participants also found that the more consumers cared about and preferred healthy eating, the more they chose green labels over (in this case) white as seemingly more healthful.

Here again, it's the same old culprit at work: lack of oversight.

There is scant oversight from governmental organizations, the FDA and FTC, over nutrition labeling. C'mon, people. FDA, FTC…USDA?

Can somebody, anybody please play on the team of the average American food consumer, who faces nationwide diabetes and obesity epidemics and is trying to make healthier selections?

But instead of regulating products already on the market, confounding consumers more and more every day, government organizations, including the FDA, are considering spending time to develop uniform front-of-package labeling.

Sure, of course, add even more labels to complicate the exceedingly simple. That seems like an efficient use of resources.

In the meantime, as they try and sort out what new label could clear up the mess that is food packaging, keep in mind that package design—and color—may be influencing your purchasing decisions.

Now that's information you can use, today, at the store, when you go to make a purchase. Yes, you're hip to the color tricks now. And as you and I have known for quite a while now, each of us needs to be our own best health advocate. May the force be with you.

4 Tricks to Keeping Fresh Produce Stocked

Staying healthy is all about setting up methods and systems.

When talking with friends, and sometimes strangers, about the biggest challenge to transitioning to healthy living, I often hear about how hard it is to keep the fridge and fruit bowl stocked when produce lasts only such a short period of time.

This makes sense. I've always noticed that if and when I am at a friend's house and a bag of Goldfish and/or greasy, kettle-cooked chips is staring me down, and within arm's reach, I will eat them.

Whereas, when I am at home, working at my desk, and all that is on hand are carrots and frozen peas and grapes and unsalted peanuts and almonds, that is what I snack on, and I am just as contented.

The biggest challenge to keeping fresh produce (especially your supergreens like kale and spinach) stocked and not wilted may be the grocery-shopping process itself, which is usually a hassle in the city (snaking lines around Trader Joe's entrances are no secret).

Still, there are a few simple strategies you can employ to help keep you on track. What I've found is, whether it's eating healthy or meeting obligations, it's all about setting up methods and systems that work for your life. Here are four to try today.

1. Order from Fresh Direct

I used to somehow always be at one New York City friend's apartment every couple of days when his fresh-food, boxed-up shipment from FD arrived. When Fresh Direct became available, it changed healthy eating at home in the city, especially for those who simply didn't have time to get to the store to pick up healthy food.

My friend worked long, tedious hours at a corporate law firm and shopping at Whole Foods or Trader Joe's just wasn't going to happen. The site solved the dilemma. It allowed him to easily pop on the site and select fruits and vegetables and other grocery items, then schedule a delivery for when he'd be home (or someone else would be around).

It's a cinch to order produce on the website, and the prices are not outrageous (we're talking arugula $1.99 each; green kale $2.29 each; and, navel oranges .99 cents each). Your produce gets delivered to your house, or office, securely packed to prevent bruising. When you go to the Vegetables tab, always click first on Produce Deals to see what's going–remember, greens wilt fast for the grocer, too. Today, escarole was $1.49 each or two for $2.00, which is a sweet savings that could add up. Go to FreshDirect.com to get started today.

2. Join A Community Garden

Another idea to try, if you live in a city, is to join a garden in your neighborhood. The rewards will not be as fast, but will come with an extra dollop of satisfaction in that you grew your own fresh food. Recently, on a weekend trip, a couple told me about meeting the man who ran a local garden near their Lower East Side apartment (I believe his name was Ernest).

They met him walking by one day, got to chatting and were soon emailing him about joining the garden and put on the wait list. Bonus: Most of these gardens have a long, dramatic New Yorkified history and story all their own, all very '80s rough-and-tumble New York. After getting on and up the waiting list, when you get the green light to join (rates are low, for this couple, $10), you get a designated plot and can plant your very own produce.

As an extra perk, you can also usually host small parties for groups of friends at the garden once you are a member, upping your coolness factor. Go to Nycgc.org or GrowNYC.org or GreenThumbNYC.org to find the community garden in your borough closest to your pad and to learn more.

3. Get Yourself A Minion (er, Task Rabbit)

Hire someone. If you work in an office, you get to a point, often, where your time is worth more money, and better spent, working rather than running errands–that's when it's time to hire a cleaning person for your a-p-t, drop your dirty clothes routinely at the corner dry cleaner's…and, yes, hire a Task Rabbit to keep your fridge and fruit bowl stocked.

This is especially your option if Fresh Direct doesn't work for you, because it doesn't allow you to give direction or because it offers the foods that you want but not at the right prices. It is now exceedingly easy to join Task Rabbit (apply in five minutes and hire your very own minion within 24 hours–often a recent college grad who is looking for extra cash and eager to please).

Your produce stocker will go to your store of choice and pick up the produce you want. You can give specific instructions (if the fresh blueberries are too high, or too ripe, go frozen; cantaloupes not too mushy; tomatoes more round and red than pink and oval) and get exactly what you want. Pay through the site and either collect bids on what someone would charge you for the service or post your own price.

Because the Task Rabbits rely on good reviews to continue getting new work, you are pretty much guaranteed to get someone who will do a good job for you. Go to TaskRabbit.com to sign up today.

4. Grocery Store Online Order and Delivery

Most grocery stores actually offer a delivery service where you can place an order and have your groceries and produce delivered to you. Shop around the neighborhood for the best prices, and know that it may take a bit of trial and error to get the right person who knows how to select the best produce for you.

Chances are, even though you're paying for the delivery, once you're stocked with fresh produce, you'll also be able to make and bring your lunch every day instead of going out to eat, which will end up saving you money. Try these two, for starters: D'agostino's or Food Emporium Delivery.

Now, the trick will be to gobble up that rainbow of produce fast once you've got the stocking covered. Consider a juicer and starting your day with some kale-celery-apple-carrot action. *Mmmm, mmm* good, a true breakfast bev of champions.

Christina Applegate Endorses FruitWater, Which Contains No Real Fruit

Christina Applegate is the buoyant, new poster gal for Coca-Cola's FruitWater, which contains no real fruit or fruit juice. A look into this and other celeb endorsements of junk food.

While listening to Pandora a short while back, through the wires came a chipper Christina Applegate letting me know that she can rel*ate* to being a busy woman trying to balance it all, and how she finds relief in FruitWater (hashtag "sparkling truth").

At the end of the ad, a male voice came on informing me that FruitWater contains no real fruit.

Wait, did I hear that correctly, I wondered?

It was hard to decipher the announcer guy's words, what with his low voice and fast-talking, garbled mumbo jumbo. Before long, the ad blasted again, and indeed, the announcer said there's no real fruit or fruit juice in the product.

On the CocaColaCompany website, I read, "The product will be available in five flavor varieties. By design it contains no fruit or fruit juice."

This is akin to having a candy bar called Chocolate Bar that contains no chocolate, or a snack called Bag 'O Nuts without one single nut inside. It's misleading, plain and simple.

Applegate, 41, is the bright, new poster face of Fruitwater, a zero-calorie, fizzy and "naturally fruit-flavored" sparkling water made by Coca-Cola's Glaceau unit (which also makes Smartwater and Vitaminwater).

The bottled drink, which hit shelves in April, is Splenda-sweetened and "enhanced with nutrients." FruitWater is being positioned as a healthier option to Coca-Cola's 16-ounce, 125-calorie, Stevia-laced Vitaminwater (the labels closely resemble one another).

Vitaminwater is that healthy-sounding beverage that provoked a lawsuit from the consumer-advocacy group Center For Science in the Public Interest, which, as a court ruled in July, can proceed as a class-action suit.

The suit claims that marketers' labels and advertising are deceptive, including claims that Vitaminwater may lower disease risk, promote healthy joints and support optimal immune function. (In 2010, Judge John Gleeson ruled that Vitaminwater's use of the word "healthy" violated FDA labeling rules, reported ABC. Sounds familiar, doesn't it?)

Sparkling...Truth?

The real "sparkling truth" is that, even though one of these has fewer calories, none of these drinks is healthy, containing any real fruits and/or vegetables, naturally synthesized antioxidants, phytonutrients, vitamins and/or minerals that research has shown can actually lower risk for disease.

These flavored waters are just gussied-up soft drinks with names that will appeal to an uninformed public trying hard to make healthier food-and-bev purchases. (By the way, sparkling-water beverages account for nearly $1 billion annually in sales.)

They're not healthy in the way that, say, a Greens For Life juice recipe from the Juice Lady Cherie Calbom is (ingredients: kale, celery, green apple, cucumber, ginger root and lemon).

Not only are they not healthy, but, as Michael F. Jacobson, executive director of CSPI told Natural News, "VitaminWater, like Coca-Cola itself, promotes weight gain, obesity, diabetes, heart disease, and cannot deliver on any of the dishonest claims it has made over the years."

Now, I feel terrible that Christina Applegate suffered from breast cancer at such a young age, and that her show *Up All Night* was canceled, but she's also a mom, and whether fair or not, from a mom I expect more.

I point out mom because at press time 17 percent of our nation's youth is obese, and since 1980, the prevalence of childhood obesity has more than doubled in children and tripled in adolescents in the United States, according to the CDC.

Not the First Time

Applegate is not the only celeb at fault, by far. This is hardly the first time a celeb took the money, shot the photo and ran.

It's reminiscent of Kim Kardashian and Brooke Burke's endorsement of those once-trendy, seemed-too-simple-to-be-true-and-were toning shoes, Skechers' Shape-ups.

The magical fitness shoes (imagine that: toned legs and nary a sweat droplet shed!) also attracted a $40 million lawsuit alleging marketers made unfounded claims.

The Federal Trade Commission concluded that Skechers had indeed lied about clinical-study findings that wearing and walking around in Shape-ups actually helped people slim down and strengthen butt, legs and stomach muscles.

Skechers denied it made false claims, but the company agreed to pay a $40 million settlement and to refund consumers who bought Skechers' Resistance Runner, Toners and Tone-ups shoes.

Even Worse: Athlete Junk-Food Endorsements

It's one thing to have screen and scene stars promoting questionable products. It's wholly another for top-tier athletes, who demonstrate peak athletic performance and ultra-conditioned physiques, to cash in by endorsing nutrient-empty, unhealthy foods and drinks, the likes of which would surely poke holes in their performance if overindulged in.

Quite a few studies in recent years have shown the influence that celeb food-and-bev endorsements have on

Americans' purchases, and by extension, their health and fitness.

Let's take a University of Liverpool research finding that celebrity endorsements of food products encourage kids to eat more of those products.

In the *Journal of Pediatrics* study, of 181 kids, from ages 8 to 11, those who had watched an ad for Walker's Crisps with English soccer pro Gary Lineker or general footage of "Match of the Day" with Lineker ate considerably more Walker's Crisps than those who watched ads for another snack or toy when offered two bowls of potato chips, one labeled Supermarket and one labeled Walker's Crisps.

Researcher Emma Boyland of the Institute of Psychology, Health and Society said in a statement, "If celebrity endorsement of HFSS (high fat salt sugar) products continues and their appearance in other contexts prompts unhealthy food intake, this would mean that the more prominent the celebrity the more detrimental the effects on children's diets."

Then there's the report released by the Rudd Center For Food Policy and Yale University, which found that the majority of the food-and-bev products endorsed by pro athletes are for unhealthy products (aka junk food).

Here, researchers analyzed 100 pro athletes and their endorsement agreements, and found that 93 percent of the beverages endorsed got their calories from added sugars and 80 percent of the food products endorsed were energy-dense and nutrient-poor.

Sports drinks comprised the largest category of celeb-endorsed products, soft drinks came in second place, and fast food in third, reported the *LA Times*.

Serena Williams's endorsements by the researchers were found to be the worst in terms of nutritional value. The group that had the most athletes endorsing food was the National Basketball Association followed by the National Football League and Major League Baseball.

Still, another study by the *European Journal of Public Health* found that cutting out unhealthy advertising targeted to kids could cut the obesity rate by up to 18 percent.

Call to Action

Social epidemiologist Abdul El-Sayed penned an open letter to LeBron James (LeBron James, Serena Williams and Peyton Manning had more food-and-bev endorsements than any other pro athletes reviewed in the Rudd/Yale report) and posted it on The 2x2 Project, a health website operated by Columbia University's Mailman School of Public Health.

The academic studied LeBron's six-year, $16 million deal with Coca-Cola and concluded that, if the beverage giant recoups its investment, this would mean 54.4 million 20-ounce Sprites sold over the course of the contract. One Sprite, by the way, contains 16 spoonfuls of sugar (my teeth hurt just typing that).

Who's Who of Celeb Endorsements

Look, this is in no way a problem to which only a few celebs have contributed. It's a societal failure. It is what happens when fame over information is prized. It is what happens when advertisements make false statements to our citizens in the face of an out-of-control obesity epidemic threatening America's health daily. It is what happens when we don't teach our children that they will be what they eat, and school curriculum doesn't include nutrition know-how to enable them to make smart, healthy choices amid a dizzying array of products calling out to them with false promises.

The ads, of course, are nothing new; but only now are they catching up with the nation. Celeb endorsements are a long tradition—you may remember these stars and the products they endorsed:

Michael Jackson (who could forget that Pepsi commercial that lit his hair on fire and resulted in second-degree scalp burns?).

Beyoncé signed a $50 million deal with Pepsi.

Peyton Manning rakes in $10 million annually from Gatorade, Wheaties, Papa John's Pizza and other brands.

Rappers Mac Miller and Lil Wayne linked with race car driver Dale Earnhardt, Jr. to endorse Mountain Dew.

The Lakers' Kobe Bryant brought in about $12 million yearly for endorsing McDonald's (remember that juicy bite into a McDonald's Big N' Tasty?).

LeBron James reportedly collected $5 million to endorse Bubblicious gum and $16 million from Coca-Cola, not to mention McDonald's.

Soccer star David Beckham endorsed Burger King smoothies.

At the end of the day, if we want to be a healthy, fit nation, we've got to disseminate correct, easily digestible information on what healthy lifestyle is and how to make the right choices every hour of every day to encourage a long, healthy and happy life.

A recent survey found that among parents with overweight kids, only 15 percent of moms and 14 percent of dads discussed healthy habits with their child. This is a discussion in which each and every one of us should engage (if you see your partner or child or friend grabbing for a mock-healthy, deceptively advertised bev, say something, because now you know), and a responsibility each and every one of us should take on.

See something, say something.

The Pros and Cons of Joining CSAs

Which are kind-of like food co-ops. Joining one gets you boxes of fresh produce, all season long.

Ask anyone who's joined a CSA what it's like, and you'll likely hear of far-out dishes made with never-heard-of veggies. Chris Mosier recalls the mouthwatering dip his wife whipped up with fava beans, olive oil and garlic scapes (garlic what?).

"Those curly, green garlic-plant tops are potent!" says Mosier. "Our breath reeked for two whole days, but that dip was so good!"

For Liran Hirschkorn, his wife's rhubarb muffins, baked from a recipe scouted online, took the prize.

Sam Meyer relished Food Network's cock-a-leekie soup he made with one week's mystery ingredient, leeks, and the punchy salsa he made with another week's, tomatillos—along with tomatoes and peppers from his share. "I never knew salsa was so easy to make," says Meyer. "Now I'm always throwing it together."

What's a CSA?

In 1995, a nonprofit called Just Food launched a sustainable food model called CSA, which stands for community-supported agriculture.

Today, there are about 100 such groups splattered throughout New York City neighborhoods (including the Bronx, Brooklyn, Manhattan and Queens) connecting the local-farmer, local-consumer dots.

You become a member by buying a share, or season's worth of produce, upfront ($400 to $600). Then you pick up a box brimming with just-picked veggies each week or two that the farmer drops in your nabe.

CSAs are a win-win. The upfront money keeps farmers afloat through the season, helping them purchase seeds and repair equipment as needed. And for members, more than just keeping their apartment kitchens bounding with fresh produce, these groups offer a way to connect with the local community, including the farmers growing their food, as well as like-minded neighbors getting creative in the kitchen.

Here's what you need to know before joining a CSA. P.S. Deadlines for winter shares are around mid-November, so get in there today if you're interested!

PRO: What in the world is that?
Each share typically contains seven to 10 types of veggies, said to be enough to feed a two- to three-person family. Some CSAs offer half-shares, catering to city dwellers who dine out religiously, or, for a few extra bucks, you can get additional shares from sister farms offering fruit, eggs, meat and even fresh flowers.

Within each batch of produce, expect a few never-seen-before veggies. Fava and cannellini beans. Tomatillos. Garlic scapes. Mosier, 33, who joined Prince George's CSA with his wife, Zhen, has received them all.

"We got stuff I'd never heard of or would try buying on my own at the store," he says. "We kept fresh vegetables in the house and also expanded our food variety and got way more inventive in the kitchen."

Along with familiar squash, radishes and eggplant, Sam Meyer, 38 and his girlfriend Bari, 43, got fennel bulbs, wax beans and chive flowers (which accent mashed potatoes marvelously, he says) at their Astoria, Queens CSA.

When Hirschkorn got rhubarb one week at his Forest Hills, Queens CSA, he scratched his head.

His wife quickly found a recipe online for rhubarb muffins that turned out scrumptious. "You can have a lot of fun trying the unique foods you get," he says, "and learning how to cook them."

CON: This ain't no delivery service.

Sorry, Dears, there's no doorstep drop-off included here. Both Mosier, who's a computer programmer, and his wife, Zhen, who works in education, commute by bike to their offices, which are not close to their distribution center.

"It was often tough getting to the pickup spot on time," he says, "and tricky transporting items home."

The couple used bike baskets and backpacks, but says pickups on the weekend or later in the evening would relieve some stress.

Meyer agrees: "It got to be a hassle to enlist friends to schlep home our veggies on our behalf. Our pickup slot was Tuesdays, 4:30 to 6:30, when my girlfriend and I had to be at work."

Before you select your group, make sure to find out what the pickup hours are. It may make more sense for you to join a distribution center closer to your office rather than your home (depending on how you plan to carry your veggie loot home.)

PRO: Save some moolah.

Ever heard of the nutritious and beloved, but pricey, Whole Foods referred to colloquially as Whole Paycheck? We certainly have. That's because shopping healthy, especially organic, isn't cheap.

Paying for a season of produce upfront by joining a CSA can save you mega dollars and cents in the long run. "The haul you lug home is dependent on the weather and crops, so some weeks are a better value than others," says Mosier. "But overall we found it to be a good bargain for the money. This year, we tried shopping the farmers' markets instead of CSA and not only ended up spending way more money, but we also didn't end up going to the market nearly as much as we thought we would, so we had way less produce around to eat."

PRO OR CON, DEPENDING: Give a little, get a lot.

"I didn't expect to like the social aspect as much as I did," says Meyer. "The chatty e-letter that listed what the current week's share would be, and members' sometimes-comic reactions to the prior week's share, along with recipe ideas, promoted a real community feeling."

Neighborhood CSA groups are run by members. As such, each member is expected to volunteer at the distribution center a few times each season. Depending of how you look at it, this could be a drag on an already airtight schedule—or it could just be a cool, new way you connect with like-minded neighbors and expand your circle (potluck dinner club, anyone?).

"We had to volunteer two shifts at the distribution center during the season," says Meyer. "I was the guy who marked off those who picked up their shares and called those who didn't show. It's easy work, and fun to meet other members."

Meyer says he also found it "cheery" to pick up the weekly veggies at the quaint local tea house that housed their distribution center.

PRO OR CON, DEPENDING: Big supply of veggies.

Hirschkorn, 32, who runs an online life insurance company (BestLifeQuote.com) and his paralegal wife joined the CSA in Forest Hills, Queens. "We got a weekly box of veggies each week, filled with more than we could eat. We'd recommend two couples split a share—or you should plan to make lots of vegetable soup."

PRO: Meet your local farmer.

Every CSA member—current or past—with whom I spoke mentioned really enjoying helping to sustain a local farmer—getting to know the farmer by name and building a relationship with the family producing their food.

"We got to meet the family whose Long Island farm the produce came from," says Hirschkorn. "Knowing we were supporting them and not some large, faceless company was rewarding."

Meyer agreed, saying he loved getting heaps of recently picked, locally grown produce each week "by a farmer whose name I knew." And, he adds, having so much colorful, fresh produce around definitely got him and his girlfriend to eat more veggies day to day. Props to that!

Before you join, here are some CSA tips:

1. Know that if you miss a week, there's no makeup time. So if you can't make a pickup, try to arrange a friend to pick up your share for you.

2. Depending on how much you eat at home each week, two couples may want to go in on a share together. Four people rotating pickup is also a mega plus.

3. The typical, most popular CSA season spans June through November, but some farmers offer winter shares, which start in early November and often span through February.

4. Check online for start dates each season. You can't join after a season has started.

5. Some CSAs have waiting periods and a limited number of people who can sign up. So expect that you may not get the first pick on your list, at least not immediately.

What Exactly Are Natural Flavors?

Not nearly as innocent as they sound.

The other day, while awaiting my train on the subway platform, I looked at the ingredients label on the juice bottle I was holding to see "natural flavors."

What is that, I wondered. The words told me nothing. I mean, could two words be any more ambiguous, mysteriously vague and non-specific?

While "natural flavors" sounded innocuous enough, certainly better-sounding than artificial flavors, such lack of transparency, such cloaks of absolute meaninglessness—when words themselves are actually rather exact—tends to incite my curiosity (read: suspicion) and send me digging.

What's A Flavor?

Let's get one thing straight from the get-go. Flavor is what gives food its taste so that it is enjoyable to eat. Flavor additives, no matter what type, whether fruit, like a yogurt's blueberry flavor or an ice cream's peach flavor, or a BBQ sauce's natural smoke flavor, have no nutritional value. Their sole purpose is to enhance taste.

"Flavors are just pure aroma chemicals, it's an aesthetic thing, to make food more palatable. There is absolutely no nutritional value in flavors," says Keith Cadwallader, PhD, a professor of food chemistry in the Department of Food Science and Human Nutrition at the University of Illinois at Urbana-Champaign.

In other words, flavors can trick us into perceiving knockoffs as the real, fresh food. But a real, freshly picked juicy peach does not need any flavor added to it to taste like peach, you see?

Most of the chemical compounds in flavors are not recognized as food by the digestive system and are not metabolized, which explains why flavors are not listed on Nutrition Facts lists.

Instead, all flavoring additives, be they natural or artificial, are manmade in laboratories by specialists called flavorists (flavorists, by the way, need not be chemists).

Flavorists mix and match chemicals in varying amounts according to recipes, or formulations, to replicate familiar flavors.

Why Do We Need Flavors—and Flavorists?

Most processed foods contain flavor additives. Why? Well, in order for people to want to buy packaged foods, to crave them, in order for processed foods to compete with deliciously tasting fresh foods, manufacturers must make their food products taste better.

An initial food purchase may be packaging-driven, writes Eric Schlosser in the book "Fast Food Nation," but subsequent purchases are based mainly on taste. You see, taste is what hooks a consumer.

Processed food without flavoring is bland food (think about green beans that have been boiling awhile compared to snap-fresh raw green beans). "The process of getting food stable—such as by heating, canning, freezing or dehydration—is detrimental to taste and changes it from what you would consider fresh," says Dr. Cadwallader. "So flavor additives offer a way to make up for the loss and goose flavor."

Take, for example, O.J. from concentrate, he adds. "You don't want to drink that stuff straight off the concentrator after it's been cooked to death. You have to add flavor—otherwise the liquid would be devoid of odor and essence."

What Is a Natural Flavor?

So, we have all come to see artificial flavors as bad, or at least the cultural perception of the word artificial has become put-back-on-the-shelf, I'm-not-feeding-my-kid-that negative.

Enter natural flavors. In short, natural flavors are an amalgamation of chemicals isolated from natural sources, whereas artificial flavors are an amalgamation of synthetic chemicals.

If you've been reading my articles, then you'll recall our old friend "natural" is quite the dietary cunundrum. When we see "natural" on packaged foods, it should raise all of our eyebrows…each and every time.

Recall the number of recent class-action lawsuits related to deceptive advertising surrounding the words "All Natural" on food labels (PepsiCo's Naked Juice, Ben & Jerry's, Snapple, Trader Joe's, etc.).

But while the label "All Natural" has never been defined and/or regulated by the FDA (explaining its rampant appearance on everything from household cleaners to cosmetics to juice bottles) and, as Robert L. Wolke, professor emeritus of chemistry, said in a *Washington Post* article, the words all natural, "can mean nearly anything the manufacturer wants them to mean or nothing at all"– the FDA actually *has* defined the words natural flavors and artificial flavors.

One Long, 100-Word Definition

Super, you might think, some clarity up in here. Well, hardly. Referred to as 21CFR101.22, and published in the Code of Federal Regulations, the definition of Natural Flavors spans more than 100 words.

As you and I have come to expect, even when needlessly complex or deceptively simple label-speak on food packaging gets decoded, its translation is just as confusing and unclear.

Alas, a natural flavor is "the essential oil, oleoresin, essence of extractive, protein hydrolysate, distillate, or any product of roasting, heating or enzymolysis, which contains the flavoring constituents derived from a spice, fruit or fruit juice, vegetable or vegetable juice, edible yeast, herb, bark, bud, root, leaf or similar plant material, meat, seafood, poultry, eggs, dairy products, or fermentation products thereof, whose significant function in food is flavoring rather than nutritional."

Got that? As Professor Wolke encouragingly summed up, "the definition plugs every possible loophole." Artificial flavors, by contrast, are those made from components (aka chemicals) not included in this definition.

Vegetarians and Vegans Beware

You read correctly that natural flavors can include animal matter (hey, they're "natural," right?). So, anyone reading "natural flavors" on an ingredients list has no way of knowing whether or not the package they are holding contains animal matter (or, for that matter, whether the "natural flavors" refer to vegetable juice, or bark, or fermentation, or yeast, etc.). Likewise, those who eat Kosher don't know whether dairy and meat mix in the food product they are holding.

Natural vs. Artificial Flavoring

Here's the deal: a person drinking an apple juice made with artificial flavors will ingest the same primary chemicals as a person drinking apple juice made with natural flavors. And neither would necessarily contain the same health benefits as, say, biting into an apple or tossing one in a juicer and gulping the resulting elixir down; though—and here's where it gets tricky—it could if, say, you were referring to the natural flavors added to V-8 juice or that cooked-to-death O.J. mentioned above.

See, food marketers, aka Big Food, know that consumers have positive reactions to the word "natural" on food packaging seeing it is synonymous with healthy or wholesome, unlike opposing words consumers assign negative meanings to, such as "artificial" and "processed."

"The truth is, the molecule is exactly the same," says Dr. Cadwallader. "Your body does not know any difference; both artificial and natural flavors are processed exactly the same way by the body."

By asking whether a packaged food contains natural or artificial flavors the average consumer's focus has shifted from the real questions at hand: Does this food have flavoring added, and if so, why?

Does it also have nutrients—like blueberries' potent superfood antioxidants, or only their flavor?

And, if not the nutrients, what's a healthier alternative with the same great (and, let's say, "real") taste? Hint: Buying and washing ripe, plump blueberries and plopping them in your plain yogurt—easy-peasy and way more healthful.

Why Such Secrecy?

The American flavor industry ropes in annual revenues upwards of $1.4 billion, according to "Fast Food Nation"'s Schlosser. Historically, the flavor industry has been quite hush-hush. There are several arguments posited as to why.

One is piracy. Formulations and recipes are not patented. Thus, if a competitor gets wind of how a flavor is produced, it can make the product, sell it for 10 cents cheaper and lure customers away, sure.

And flavors are complex. Take the flavor and aroma of coffee.

It contains more than 800 chemical compounds. While the flavorists' version would contain way fewer (the fewer chemicals one can use to get the taste gist right, the cheaper to produce and better for the manufacturer) there would still be a long list of unrecognizable chemical names on the product if listing the specifics of a natural flavor was required, deterring and confusing consumers even more.

Then there is another reason manufacturers prefer not to mention what's behind natural flavors: The primary source of the natural flavor may be unpleasant and unsavory to read or think about, the last thing you'd want to see listed on a food item.

Say, castoreum. While most consumers would not know offhand what that is, Google would quickly illuminate for them that it is the chemical compound beavers use to mark their territory. Because of the types of leaves and bark beavers eat, this brown sludge is vanilla-scented.

But wait, it gets worse. Due to the location of the sacs that deposit the slime—near the anal glands—the liquid is usually a mixture of urine, anal-gland secretions and castor-gland secretions, reports an article in *Time*. Yum!

An *International Journal of Toxicology* found that manufacturers have been using castoreum heavily in perfumes—and foods—for years.

Now, castoreum may be OK for your scented desk candle (*may* be), but it's doubtful there's room for it on the dessert table. Castoreum is just one example of an item that could appear on an ingredient label under the generic umbrella term "Natural Flavors."

Takeaways

The going assumption is that most American consumers are lazy. That they don't care, or want to know. They like taste, buy for taste, are addicted to taste and will overlook anything to get more of it.

But some of us (ahem) do not believe this. There is one easy way to avoid confusion: keep your food simple—"real" simple.

Eat the real, whole fruit or vegetable whenever possible and you never have to fret about where the flavors contained within came from.

Buy plain (unflavored) yogurt and add real fruit (real is the new natural).

If you buy frozen berries—and remember, frozen produce maintains all of its good-for-you nutrients—make sure that the ingredients lists contain nothing but the berries themselves.

Buy pure vanilla extract and you won't have to puzzle over whether the imitation kind you're holding, made with "natural flavors," contains unsavory, mystery spurts.

I know, I know, we have been conditioned to believe that buying produce and making our own food is time-consuming and tedious. We're too busy for that. Nonsense!

I've been experimenting and am here to tell you that that is just not true. The key is keeping fresh produce stocked. And that's just strategy. Chopping up tomatoes to make fresh spaghetti sauce, or salsa, or rinsing and tossing berries into your oatmeal, yogurt or blender to make a vitality juice takes maybe five to 10 minutes.

The taste, not to mention the nutrients, can't be beat. Why throw away one meal—when every food you put in your mouth could work in your favor, and actually benefit you? Key takeaway: Real is the new natural. Spread the word.

Lady Gaga's Waist on Glamour Cover Is Not Humanly Possible

Lady Gaga's too-thin waist on her Glamour *magazine cover is highly disturbing. It sends a dangerous wrong (and unhealthy) message to readers—especially young girls who are at risk for developing eating disorders.*

It's that time of year when we celebrate abundance, joining at the table with family and friends to break bread together and celebrate the autumn season's plentiful harvest, sharing blessings large and small.

And as you were plunking down all the chunky stuffing and creamy-pumpkin-pie ingredients on the conveyer belt, you probably looked up to see, front and center, a *Glamour* magazine cover featuring a subhuman, sickly thin cinched waist, squeezed between two tiny hands.

That'd be the way-too-tiny-to-be-humanly-possible waist of cover girl Lady Gaga. Suddenly all the festive holiday recipes and indulgent ingredients and meal plans seem guilty. And that's just plain disgraceful.

Media images of women with disturbingly waif-thin waists are nothing new, sadly. We have come to expect this from fashion magazines. But *Glamour*, and its audience, had been decidedly different.

In a more embracing girlfriend-y tone, it covered heady topics with reporting and research by and for smart women alongside lighter topics. Each month it also featured extensive confidence-boosting and totem-rising advice for careeristas.

And, yet. The typical response to these larger-than-life, too-thin cover images of drastically unrealistic and impossible proportions is, "Horrible, yes, but we all know these images are Photoshopped and manipulated to look that way."

Not so fast with the dismissal. While that may be true for those of us who have matured (read: aged) into adults, the disheartening, overlooked fact is that the target demographic for these magazines is often younger. Way younger.

In fact, they speak to young women who are likely at the pinnacle of a common adolescent struggle with body image, many who may be on the brink of tipping into the eating disorder category.

For these impressionable girls, a national magazine's cover not only signals approval of, but aspiration to, being rail thin. Thus, using such snapshots as a cover photo is an especially damaging decision. Shame on those whose desks this passed.

In the U.S., 20 million women and 10 million men battle a clinically significant eating disorder at some time in their life, according to the National Eating Disorder Association.

What's more, a surprising for-all-the-wrong-reasons 2012 study in the *Journal of Eating Disorders* found that an increasing number of older women are battling food issues, and some 13 percent of women ages 50-plus display symptoms of eating disorders (to put that in perspective, breast cancer affects about 12 percent of this group).

How Did This Cover Photo Come to Be?

We would hope in 2013, when a record-breaking four in 10 households with kids under 18 have a woman as the confident, successful sole or primary breadwinner, we would not have to remind media decision makers of the power of their selections—and the responsibility that goes along with that position.

Even high-profile women, such as Ariana Huffington, coming out to the public about their own daughters' struggles with eating disorders in order to make us all more aware, have obviously not heightened the media's sensibilities.

Color us shocked, but somehow, a whole editorial team of people looked at this photo circulating around the office and signed off their approval.

It is important to point out how it typically works at magazines: Cover photos are stapled to large galley folders and circulated to an entire list of media professionals on staff, from editor-in-chief to executive and deputy editors, to art directors and photo editors, to copy editors and fact-checkers for their initials and signatures, and iterations of the tremendously important cover image circulate at least two, if not three, times.

And this Lady Gaga photo was signed off, and "approved," for November, aka the Thanksgiving feast month.

Is This Waist Humanly Possible?

So, could this waist possibly be for reals? "Absolutely not," says Marjorie Nolan Cohn, MS, RD, CDN, who is a national spokesperson for the Academy of Nutrition & Dietetics. "The image appears to be significantly Photoshopped. There is another photo of Lady Gaga at the *Glamour* cover event, and her thumbs don't nearly wrap around her waist the way they did on the cover."

So What Is a Healthy Weight?

With so many false images of what a woman's waist is supposed to ideally look like, how is a young woman (or man) supposed to know what her healthy weight range is?

Good question. In clinical settings, a person's healthy weight range is determined by using body mass index (BMI) along with weight history, diet history, a physical assessment and laboratory values, explains Gina Neill, MS, RD/LDN, dietician and founder of Glow Nutrition.

BMI, which gauges healthy weight range based on height, is calculated this way: square your height in inches, divide your weight in pounds by your height squared, and multiply that number by 703. (Make sure to measure your "current" height, because over the years our height can change and be less than we remember, or even what's listed on our driver's license).

Less than 18.5 is considered underweight; healthy weight is considered between 18.5 and 24.9; overweight is considered 25 to 29.9; and obese is considered 30 or more, explains Lisa Young, PhD, RD/CDN, who is an adjunct nutrition professor at NYU in the Department of Nutrition, Food Studies and Public Health.

Is This Damaging to the Public?

Abso-frickin-lutely. Or, as Jennifer Lombardi, executive director of the Eating Recovery Center of California says, yes. She should know.

Lombardi's five-year struggle with anorexia began at age 17, though she admits to first beginning to wrestle with disordered eating and exercise abuse around age 11.

"Like so many young adolescent girls going through puberty, I was uncomfortable in my ever-changing body and dabbled in diet pill use, bouts of extreme exercise and numerous fad diets," she says.

During her eating disorder, Lombardi admits she would have idolized how Lady Gaga looks on *Glamour*'s cover and how any celebrity or model looked on the cover of a magazine.

"I knew that most likely the image had been airbrushed, but I didn't care. I was so driven to look and be a certain way that I would have done anything to 'achieve the unachievable.' Common sense and logic took a backseat to perfectionism and the painful drive to achieve it."

Looking at images like this now, says Lombardi, makes her sad. "Despite all that we know about how these images negatively impact self-esteem and put forth unrealistic body expectations (both stated and implied), they continue to occur.

My worry is how this not only impacts individuals who are at risk for developing eating disorders, but for countless others who struggle with subclinical disordered eating and go to extremes in the pursuit of an unrealistic, thin ideal."

What Is Being Underweight?

"Body mass index, BMI, is commonly used to determine if one is underweight," says Dr. Young.

"If a person has too little body fat, or if a woman does not get her period, these could be signs of being underweight." Potential warning signs of an eating disorder include a preoccupation with food, irritability and excessive exercise, Dr. Young adds. "These are signs of a potential eating disorder. An evaluation with a health professional is warranted."

If you are concerned that a loved one may be battling a food issue, Lombardi suggests these action steps:

1) Write down all the things that you notice and are concerned with (for example, make a list of behaviors you've witnessed and/or changes in a person's mood).

2) Learn more about eating disorders (check out the National Eating Disorders Association and Eating Recovery Center's online resources) and treatment options in your area (a valuable resource for treatment referrals is EdReferral.com).

3) Finally, set aside time to speak directly to your loved one. Eliminate all distractions (cell phones, TV, etc.) and be

clear. "You might start off by telling the person how much you care about them, and then clearly state the reasons why you are concerned. Encourage him/her to, at the very least, seek out an assessment from a professional who specializes in eating disorder treatment," says Lombardi. Offering to go with a loved one to the appointment can sometimes help, she adds.

I hope you all savored each and every bite of your delicious turkey dinner on Thanksgiving, without one dollop of doubt or guilt.

I'll tell you why. An interesting finding in the journal *Perception* concluded that men find female bodies more attractive in winter months (yes, referring to our voluptuous curves). Researchers believe that a contrast effect may be the cause, according to Oprah.com, and that in winter, the attractiveness criteria changes as men are exposed to more heavily clothed women. So gobble up, my dears, and enjoy. Survey says, you look ravishing!

Real Salad! Fresh Salad! In A Vending Machine!

It's happened and may soon becoming to a shopping mall near you.

The age-old vending machine just got a fresh, sexy makeover—not to mention a noble new purpose.

It's all thanks to an innovative little food company with a big idea called Farmer's Fridge. Founder Luke Saunders, 27, had the brilliant concept of offering healthy, daily-made salads right out of a refrigerated vending machine. Yep, those leafy, green machines—good-for-you real food—can now be out-of-a-machine convenient, too!

Where the Revolution Started

Just six weeks after launching its first-ever refrigerated vending machine in the Chicago-based Garvey food court, urged on by popular demand, the food company has now opened its second automated salad seller at the Lake Forest Tollway.

OK, easy there, New Yorkers. I know we're used to being health-innovative first adopters. We're next on the list, according to Saunders. "We really want to be there," says Saunders, who's originally from Basking Ridge, New Jersey.

The company strategically put its first machine in downtown Chicago—in a food court—where there were no other healthy food options. And, as the company had hoped, the shoppers gobbled up the goodness. "The response has been amazing!," says Saunders.

What's on Offer?

With gourmet salad options like The Free-Radical Assassin (mixed greens, goat cheese, mixed berries, almonds, carrots, sprouts and flaxseed with white balsamic vinaigrette), The High Protein Salad (spinach, corn, peas, pumpkins seeds, figs, broccoli, chickpeas, shredded Parmesan and quinoa with a lemon tahini dressing) and The Mediterranean Salad (mixed greens, artichoke hearts, cannellini beans, organic cucumber, tomato, kalamata olives, Parmesan, pine nuts and oregano with a red-wine vinaigrette), how could they not eat up?

The agenda here is offering foods packed with organic, local, nutrient-rich ingredients in environmentally friendly BPA-free plastic jars (hmm, transparent? we like that concept).

Just grab a fork and go. Plus, the layered, stacked salad-prep technique guards against sogginess, keeping the fruits, vegetables, grains, nuts, seeds and other ingredients crisp and vibrant.

How Does It Work?

Thought it couldn't be done? Well, Saunders saw a massive gap in the food industry. While traveling and on the go, his gut told him he wasn't the only one craving healthier "fast-food" options. With his strong manufacturing background, Saunders put two and two together and realized making this much-needed concept a reality wasn't rocket science.

"No one had connected the food and vending and fabrication dots." The entrepreneur says he was thinking on the idea for two years, while his wife pursued her career as a lawyer.

In the end, it just came down to stellar time management, or what I like to call methods and systems. Each weekday, a small crew gathers at 5 a.m. to chop up and package the produce, whipping up salads, nutritious snacks and breakfast bites. (Well, it took smarts, too, to understand that layering the food would keep it fresh, and that the lowest acidity items had to be on bottom, etc.)

The goods are delivered and loaded into the machines around 9 a.m. Whatever's still there the next morning goes to local food banks (hmm, did they get that idea from another of my fave "fresh" enterprises, Pret A Manger?) "It's just part of the morning delivery route," says Saunders.

The company's linked arms with SPE, a certification company, to ensure high quality in its food offerings, which contain whole grains, veggies and lean proteins. Want even more of a protein punch with your salad? Easily add chicken, tuna or salmon.

"There's a reason nobody's done this before," says Saunders. "It's really challenging, getting the operations part down." Still, Saunders seems to have figured it out.

The best part? You can get a protein-packed salad for $7 (and yes, Dears, plastic is accepted).

Going by ever-popular Just Salad's prices, where one salad can easily put you back two digits, or those airport iceburg-lettuce salads, typically running at least $10 and not mason-jar-layered fresh, that's a real steal. (*Psst*, hit the vending machine after 6 p.m., and you'll get a $1 discount). All around genius, we say! Um, so can you plug one into our building pronto, please? And everyone working on the team, I hope you've negotiated a fat chunk of stock options (big wink).

HelloFresh Makes Anyone A Gourmet Health Chef

Meal-prep delivery services take the guesswork out of the healthy-eating equation.

As you know, I'm always on the lookout for innovative, newfangled tools that make healthy lifestyle more achievable for everyone.

When I heard about the meal-prep start-up called HelloFresh, of course I had to give the concept a whirl.

What It Is

HelloFresh launched in London in early 2012. Ed Boyes had this cool idea of having chefs create original, healthy recipes and then assembling all the ingredients, precisely portioned out for the dishes, and shipping directly to consumers' doorsteps.

Since its arrival, the start-up has been on the up and up. Just in September 2013 alone, HelloFresh attracted $7.5 million in venture capitol funding from Russia's Phenomen Ventures (also an early investor in Fab.com). Keeping his word, CEO Dominik Richter used the money to expand to the U.S.

How It Works

Each week, chefs design new, original recipes, collaborating with Michelin star restaurant Aquavit. Then, subscribers browse and select from each week's recipe menu—not just any recipes but healthy, nutritious recipes.

The three meals I sampled included ingredients such as Greek yogurt, fresh arugula, garlic and onion, along with health-promoting spices such as Indian-inspired cardamom and turmeric.

So you select a recipe, and delivered to your doorstep will be a padded, ice-pack-cooled box, loaded with laminated, simple recipes (we're talking five steps or less) and all of their associated ingredients, which are bagged, labeled and perfectly proportioned for each recipe.

Pro: Generous Portions

At first, looking at the individually wrapped ingredients, I was skeptical that there was enough food for two people (hey, my man, like most men, likes a hearty meal).

But when my guy and I cooked two of the dishes together, we were pleased to see that each meal provided enough food to satiate us both. While this means no leftovers for lunch, it also means no waste. And HelloFresh says that typically 40 percent of our food is wasted.

Pro: Healthy, Farm-Fresh Ingredients

One of my personal favorite go-to ingredients is fresh ginger. Now, I was not asked what I wanted to try, but was just sent three sample, standard meal preps.

How pleased was I to discover that each recipe included fresh ginger, along with other faves like garlic, onion and fresh herbs and spices—not to mention nonflavored Greek yogurt. It was very clear to me that whoever is putting together these recipes places good-for-you ingredients at the core of the menu.

Con: It's a Time Commitment

These aren't 10-minute, grab-and-go recipes. And while you won't have to shop—and endure the hassles of traveling and line waiting—you will actually have to cook.

Maybe we're slow in the kitchen, but while each recipe was supposed to take us 30 minutes or less, each took us more like 50 minutes from prep to plate. One of the chicken recipes even had me trimming fat from the bird, which was something new to me and a bit more intensive than I expected.

But I can see how this would appeal to people who really enjoy cooking and want to be involved in preparing the food they are eating, handling the ingredients, peeling, mixing and chopping.

If you're more of a rip open bag; dump; and, eat type, this isn't for you. If you're a couple who enjoys whipping up your dinner together over a glass of wine after a long day, then done! Date night to your doorstep.

Con: You Do the Dishes

Obviously, when you come home from work exhausted and place a call to your fave neighborhood restaurant, your dinner also arrives on your doorstep…all hot and prepared for you, complete with utensils and containers you can just use and toss.

Yes, this is wasteful and we'd rather not go this route, but we all know there are those nights when you're just too tired to care. You just don't want to lift another finger to prepare food—or clean the dishes afterward!

Pro: You'll Learn to Cook ... Seamlessly

If your New Year's resolution involves learning how to prepare your own healthy meals at home, you'd no doubt greatly benefit from trying out a nutritious meal-prep service like HelloFresh.

That's because you get to keep the easy-to-follow, slickly laminated and designed recipes. Just by following the recipes you will start to see what healthy ingredients health nuts routinely buy and have around (hint: think garlic, onion and lemon juice).

Once you have the recipes, you don't necessarily need to keep buying the delivered ingredients. You with me here? These recipes are so simple and clear, they really can turn anyone into a healthy cook.

Con: It Ain't Cheap

As with many health-boosting, convenience-minded services, ordering a recipe/ingredient box from HelloFresh will set you back a shiny penny.

So, here's what you need to know. While the website will tell you meals start from $11, and they do, at the moment, you have to order a minimum of three meals together, which will arrive packaged in one large box.

Boxes are for two or four people, with or without meat, delivered each Wednesday or Thursday (depending on which of the participating 30 states you're in).

The least you'll spend is $59 for a two-person veggie box. From there, $69 for a two-person classic box, $109 for a four-person veggie and $129 for a four-person classic.

As with all spending, it's all about the comparisons. If you'd otherwise be dining out or ordering out and tacking on tips, you may save. However, if you're used to buying and pricing out healthy ingredients, then you may be spending more. For example, one of the ingredients in one of our meals was a can of Goya garbanzo beans.

Now, what came to my mind? Well, if you know a bit about health, a bit about food shopping, and the sport of saving money, you know that beans are one of the most underrated superfoods out there, and cans of Goya beans are quite cheap. It's worth pointing out, though, that our three meals also came with fresh chicken, shrimp and beef.

Tip: while there is no minimum requirement for subscriptions, you must give one week's notice if you want to stop receiving boxes.

Hey, I'm all for trying new things, but don't take my word for it. If a healthy lifestyle is something you're striving to get closer to this year, a meal-prep delivery service like HelloFresh, or one of its competitors (like Blue Apron or Fresh Dish), is certainly worth a try.

A Look at the Phrase, "You Look Great, Have You Lost Weight?"

Should commenting on a person's weight be off limits?

It always catches me by surprise when I run into a person I haven't seen in a while and they comment on my physical appearance. Whether it's a new haircut or shoes, it always astonishes me. And the weight question, to me, always seemed in a league of its own.

Every time I hear the ol' "You look great! Have you lost weight?," I think, how *dare* you comment on my, or his, or her, weight? Well, maybe I'm the oddball here, because I hear it all the time—so the line I see must be drawn in sand.

Issues, Issues Everywhere

Much of my reaction has to do with my work, and my life experience. In high school, I knew many girls who had trouble with food and eating and weight. As young girls, we didn't recognize what we were seeing and hearing at the time for what it was. Yet, the signs were everywhere.

Everyone knew *some* girl whose father commented on her weight that one time on the soccer field, thereby triggering years of weight battles. And everyone knew *some* girl who had a bag of pretzels and a diet soda for lunch every day. And everyone knew *some* girl whose period mysteriously stopped. Or *some* girl who oddly stripped off all the cheese from her pizza slice before eating it.

I wouldn't understand the full magnitude of what I had seen until years later, when struggles were made public and reporting and research enlightened me.

Recently in my work, I was talking with a woman who'd been treated for compulsive exercise. She told me how confusing it had been to her during a time when, in private, she was obsessing over weight and torturing her body, yet in public, people were raving about how amazing she looked. "You look great!" they'd say.

Even though she knew her motivations and actions were destructive, in her mind, which she'd be the first to admit was warped at the time, these comments would give her the OK to proceed. "Even if the tactics are harsh, they must be working, right?" she'd think.

Oh God, I thought. Have I uttered such things before and unknowingly sent a privately suffering person into a tailspin of confusion, possibly even propelling their disastrous self-abuse?!

Why Do We Say It?

Admittedly, I was ready to stricken the phrase from my chitchat arsenal for life. But it's not so black and white, as Adam Silberstein, Psy.D, an LA-based clinical psychologist, rapidly points out.

"If somebody looks good, our culture gives permission to say, 'You look good,'" he says, "and if a profound shift in weight occurs, which is very visible, people acknowledge it."

Social Context Matters

Really, the social context determines the appropriateness of the question, says Don Lynch, PhD, a professor of psychology at Maine's Unity College.

In fact, it's key.

Think about it. In the context of a physical exam by your physician, of course asking about weight is appropriate, says Dr. Lynch. And the phrase is often thrown out during chance encounters with people we don't know well. All the examples that came to my mind were such. You bump into an acquaintance unexpectedly, whom you haven't seen in a while. It's small talk.

"When you run into someone, from a cultural standpoint you want to say something positive—'like your new haircut … glasses … or, look … fill in the blank,'" says Art Markman, PhD, professor of psychology and marketing at the University of Texas at Austin, who also wrote *Smart Thinking.*

Whereas, with our closest friends, we typically know the hot buttons or struggles close to home, he explains, and thus, which topics should be covered with sensitivity and care.

We're Not Mind Readers

And that's just it—in most people's minds they're saying something positive.

"When people remark on appearance," says Dr. Silberstein, "it is not in the spirit of ill intentions. Is it up to every adult in the U.S. to have an awareness of eating disorders?"

Dr. Markman agrees and points out that nobody would ever say, "Wow, you got huge. What happened?"

True, and you just think for a hot second how miffed and vocal I would become if I heard some semblance of that phrase mumbled to anyone around me, stranger or not.

"The complimenter can't know an acquaintance's psychic makeup and it's unfair to think the responsibility of awareness of issues lies with the individual commenting," adds Dr. Silberstein.

"We generally don't *not* acknowledge something because it could be a sensitive issue, for example not mention alcohol or gambling because the person we're talking with may have an addiction."

Ah, phew. This largely takes the guilt off the shoulders of the world's awkward (or careless) blurter-outers. But now what?

Avoidance Isn't the Answer

Acknowledgement of the obvious shouldn't be condemned, says Dr. Silberstein.

As a former food addict who once weighed 300 pounds, Dr. Silberstein, who is also the co-founder of The Source Health and Wellness Treatment Center, never expected people not to comment after he shed 130 pounds. He actually had a different negative reaction with which to contend.

"If someone is on a new healthy path, or routine, trying to reach a healthy goal weight, they can hear this and think, 'Hey, I'm there, I can stop now, go back to how I used to eat.'"

For him, he'd hear inspiration, but it would also sound like graduation day, and thus make it harder to stick to his healthy regimen. He admits the primary distortion was his, saying, "It was not about body size for me, but my relationship with food—that was the most important piece for me to accept."

What you Hear Is What You Get

So there's intention, and then there's perception. If a person hears such a question ("Have you lost weight?") as permission to continue on his or her destructive path, that is the listener's perception, and in that case, distortion.

"If I am a compulsive overeater and then starve myself to lose weight, I may use this comment to service that part of me that is not healthy," says Dr. Silberstein.

"But while the listener is responsible, it is important to keep in mind that the listener may not be aware of their own vicious thought cycle because he or she is suffering. The most important thing is that if someone has a destructive response, then that person may be suffering."

Context With a Dose of Culture

Context, yes, but let's not forget our wacky, obsessed culture. "We Americans are obsessed with concerns of being overweight," says Dr. Lynch, "and there is also a pervasive cultural obsession with physical appearance, as evidenced by the media's emphasis on Madison Avenue images of sexual attraction and physical beauty."

Frankly, he's not sure why so many of us tend to frame a comment about a person's appearance into a question about weight. "I can see how people might take offense to a question about their body weight," he adds. (Hear, hear, Prof!)

"Europeans," he says, "do indeed take offense to someone asking about their weight and instead prefer favorable comments about personal appearance, demeanor or affect."

In the End

Well, I like Europe. And Europeans. Quite a bit, actually. And the thing is, I do have an awareness. Big time (and now, so do you, Dears). What's more, my eyes can see way more than a person's body.

So while the burden of the blurter-outer has largely been erased here in this space, the next time you see me you can expect me to say, "Hey, you look fabulous!" and as you stare at me waiting, searchingly, perhaps wanting desperately, I'll slyly add, "and I am so happy to see *You*."

Exercising to Death

Compulsive exercisers just can t stop, getting way too much of a good thing.

Wendy Greene was severely depleted. She'd just banged out an excruciating hourlong workout, her third of the day, her poor, weak body pushed to perform on a measly 1,000 calories a day. She got in her car, began driving. In a flash, her tired limbs and frame gave out at a downtown Denver intersection. She faded away. All went dark. Only a miracle can explain how she ended up at a stop light when the blackout struck. Had she nodded off a moment before, or after, she could have died.

Greene, now 30, says the event shook her up but ultimately seemed par for the course. It would take three more years for Greene to seek treatment for compulsive exercise — by then, severely isolated, unable to concentrate on, or finish, anything, unable to perform her physically demanding job as a firefighter … and exercising herself to death. "Life," she says, "started falling apart. I made bad decisions … romantic, financial. I just couldn't think clearly."

What Is Obsessive Exercise

Compulsive exercise, obsessive exercise, exercise bulimia — it goes by different terms, explains Jennifer Sommer, MS, RD, CSSD, a registered dietitian at the Denver-based Eating Recovery Center, who treats this lesser-known form of the bulimia eating disorder, in which a person is addicted to exercise and cannot stop on their own. The method of purging is exercise. It's tough to identify because generally exercise is beneficial, and this purging happens in the open, not like sneaky vomiting or laxative downing behind closed doors.

"I don't like the term 'excessive exercise,' because it's not necessarily doing too much exercise," says Sommer, "but exercising for the wrong reasons — not for health or to train for a race, but solely to control weight and shape or as a punishment for eating bad foods."

Compulsive exercise could occur even when a person works out the recommended 30 minutes a day, most days of the week. It becomes problematic when, for example, a day is ruined if a workout is missed, or one never takes a day off, even when sick or injured, or one repeatedly cancels social plans to work out. Exercise becomes the top priority, significantly harming relationships and causing physical injuries.

Compulsive exercise is especially problematic during the holidays, says Sommer, as treats-loaded parties abound and gym sessions become a way to compensate for negative feelings about indulging.

How It Starts

Often, compulsive exercise starts with healthy intentions. One exercises for pleasure, or stress relief, or the endorphin rush, or just to feel better. Over time, one has to do more to get the same positive boost. Before long, it's never enough. Exercise starts ruling life.

"It's not uncommon for obsessive exercisers to join multiple gyms, so as not to be discovered," says Sommer. "Anytime you have someone doing something in secrecy, they know they're overdoing it."

Dangerous Consequences

Overexercising takes a physical and mental toll. "Physical injuries include strains, sprains, stress fractures, osteoporosis, arthritis, and overexercising can make body fat too low and a person dangerously underweight" says Sommer. "If for any reason they can't get their workout in, it can lead to extreme anxiety and/or purging. It's an extremely slippery slope." It can also lead to anxiety and depression, and, for women, amenorrhea, or loss of three consecutive periods.

Personal Trainers' Roles

We've all been in that class, when you spot a gymgoer near you looking frail, tired and weak. Too weak to be in a highly intensively workout class. Throughout the class, you worry about them, hope they'll be okay. Why does the gym allow this? Why doesn't the instructor say something? Is this sweet, little thing going to pass out next to me, and if so, what should I be prepared to do?

Pointing fingers isn't the answer. Personal trainers don't receive training on how to spot compulsive exercisers or eating disorders, says Jodi Rubin, a certified eating disorder therapist of 15 years who founded Destructively Fit, which offers training courses online and at gyms to help fitness pros identify and address these issues. Fitness pros have told her they saw the physical symptoms, but didn't know how to approach people they were concerned about. Ironically, compulsive exercise is also quite common among fitness pros. Many reached out to me while I was working on this story. In fact, an obsession of sorts could be what brought trainers and instructors to the industry, says Rubin.

Causes

Often the cues for compulsive exercise are external, says Rubin. "The pressure, the images out there point to spending more time at the gym in pursuit of completely unrealistic goals. We see these emaciated models presented as beautiful. And a lot of fitness stuff sends the same messages — ads for gyms, social media displays, etc."

But there has to be an emotional vulnerability there, to take these cues and use them against yourself, adds Rubin. "At root, often there's self-esteem trouble. People think, 'I feel terrible on the inside, and I can't control it, but I can control the outside and make that look good.' It's a dangerous cycle."

Greene, now a full-time nursing student in Wyoming, is getting life back on track. Still, despite counselors' advice to walk away from CrossFit, she continues to coach it. "I need the endorphins," she says. "[As a coach] I can spot it a mile away," she says. "CrossFit is intense. They disregard safety, continue moving with elevated heart rates, go pale," she says of compulsive exercisers in her classes. "They must compete, but can't catch their breath. They'll take a week or two to recover … and then come back. It is really scary."

Where "Members-Only" Means 50-Plus Pound Overweight

A gym where everybody knows your name, and your struggle.

For Brianne Angus, it was one nasty comment too many, and one that would change her life.

It had been two years since she'd seen a male colleague, who'd been transferred to another office. During that time, she had ballooned to 297 pounds. When the two bumped into one other, the guy, who used to whistle at and flirt with her, now eyed her with disgust.

Looking her up and down, judgingly, he said, as if he just couldn't help himself, "I thought the belly was supposed to leave after the baby," and walked off.

Utterly humiliated, Angus scrambled back to her desk and tried hard not to cry. But there was no reserve of confidence to draw from to feel better. She felt beaten down. On that day, she decided to never let anybody make her feel like that again. She knew change was needed.

"On the outside, I'd handle that kinda stuff with humor, saying, 'Yep, watch me go eat my burger!' But really, it hurt. You know you're overweight. It's no surprise. It's a daily, visible struggle."

Today, the 31-year-old mother of two is general manager (and franchise owner) at Canada's first Downsize Fitness, located in Ontario. It's a gym with one unique requirement. Anyone who wants to join this fitness club must be at least 50 pounds overweight according to their personal BMI.

What It Is

Downsize Fitness began in Chicago (wow, Chicago is really competing with New York, here, as a first adopter), opening its first franchise in 2011. Founder Francis Wisniewski was 360 pounds at the time, and had battled with his weight his entire life. He wouldn't go near any gym for fear of ridicule.

Instead, he opened his own ... where everyone had to be just like him, overweight. The franchise took off quickly, and now has two locations in Texas (Dallas and Fort Worth) and two in Illinois (Chicago and Naperville). Just this month, Angus opened her location in Ontario, and has attracted some 70 members. All told, the U.S. gyms have lured hundreds of members, ranging in weight from 200 to 700 pounds. And together, this crew is shedding mountains. Combined, U.S. members have shed some 5,500 pounds. Downsize President Kishan Shah, formerly a private equity investor at Goldman Sachs, was 400 pounds when he first joined the gym. Now, he's half that size.

The Big Idea

The concept, of acceptance and a shared weight-loss journey, is the antithesis of what American viewers see on television shows such as *The Biggest Loser* (I mean, really, just think for a hot second about the play on words there). This decidedly different approach is one that will serve those trying to lose weight better than any such ratings-topper shows.

That's because it turns out that what people could really use, to help them shed pounds, is encouragement and support, not a drill sergeant.

A recent University of Alberta study found that watching competitors scream, cry, vomit and wince their way through strenuous workouts was more likely to turn viewers off and create negative attitudes toward exercise than to motivate them in their own weight-loss efforts.

No matter the study participants' weight or fitness level, the thoughts they wrote down after watching *The Biggest Loser* clips were more negative than thoughts written down after watching *American Idol* (which also involves a fair bit of sweat).

"People are screaming and crying and throwing up, and if you're not a regular exerciser you might think this is what exercise is," said lead researcher Tanya Berry, PhD, Canada's Research Chair in Physical Activity Promotion. "That it's this horrible experience where you have to push yourself to the extremes and the limits, which is completely wrong."

How It's Different

At Downsize Fitness, all classes are low-impact and most personal trainers hired have themselves triumphed over personal weight-loss battles. What's more, certain locations such as Angus's also offer access to on-site nutritionists and meal plans.

Downside also offers tinted windows, equipment (ellipticals, treadmills and stationary bikes) tailored to the heavyset (thicker cushions, wider seats), and you'd be hard-pressed to find any mirrors.

Walls are lined instead with inspiring before-and-after photos of members who've, well, downsized significantly. People with heart conditions are required to supply their own Polar heart monitor.

"I like to tell my members, 'If you're moving, your body is burning,'" says Angus. "And you are miles ahead of the person still stuck on the couch, watching TV. I tell my members, 'You're my people.'"

There's a lot of personal attention doled out, as well. Instead of trainers barking at members to push harder, here trainers carry a different tune.

"We're not having members bounce around and try things that are impossible for where they're at. It's more like every two minutes, we're reminding them to drink water or take a break. We grow together."

There are 15-minute windows between classes to gain feedback from members, and if you don't show for a few days, expect a check-in call, text or Facebook ping from

Angus or one of her colleagues to find out where you've been.

"This isn't *Biggest Loser.* It's low-impact, designed for fun and effectiveness," says Angus. "It's about feeling good and getting healthy, not about getting skinny."

In the spring, she plans to start a members-only softball team.

How Much Does It Cost?

There are two main Downsize Fitness packages, explains Angus. The first, an eight-class bundle with semi-personal training and nutritionist access costs $149 per month; the second, including unlimited classes plus seminars and home video access to classes, costs $229 per month.

Stigma, Real or Imagined?

But is the ridicule that overweight people talk about experiencing at gyms real or imagined? I've often found that everyone at the gym around me is focused on their own improvement and too consumed with their own performance and progress to notice others' forms. But whether the insecurity comes from the inside or surroundings is beside the point, says Angus.

"The reality is that for me, and people like me, gyms presented discomfort," she says.

"If I stepped into one, I'd be pulling at my clothes the whole time, and sure that other people were staring at me. I'd just be uncomfortable," says Angus, adding that to her, gyms were places fit people went to get more fit. "Society has made overweight people feel uncomfortable and unwelcome, wherever they go," she adds.

How's It Going?

"Success!" exclaims Angus, recalling one member who, when she joined, watched her first Zumba class from a chair, and who, just last week, actually participated in and completed her first 45-minute class. "I was so happy for her. I wanted to go and buy pom-poms," said Angus with infectious pride.

I've Lost Weight, Now What?

So, do you quit when you reach your goal and sweat off that excess 50 pounds? No, says Angus, you can stick around and become a mentor for new members and/or become a trainer. In fact, many recent hires are vets of the gym who had reached their fitness goals.

Trending Now

We've seen this type of open-arms "come one, come all" encouragement from a few other gyms recently, points out NPR, with Planet Fitness's "judgment-free zone" and Omaha, Neb.'s Square One gyms, swearing members won't be surrounded by any "size 2s sprinting on treadmills."

And have you seen those gorgeous New York City subway ads for the YMCA ("Be You. Join the Y."), complete with real people's smiling, rosy-cheeked faces?

Well done, I say. A big first step to paring down America's obesity epidemic is getting folks into the gym, which of course means making them feel comfortable and welcome.

Acknowledgements

These essays first appeared on the New York startup website, TheBlot.com, which launched in 2013. I am grateful to have had a place where I could write about what irked me, intrigued me, made me happy, and made me sad with no rewrites, only a few tiny proofreading tweaks and no meddling at all in my true voice, my true message and the authentic copy that poured out of me. I am grateful to so many of the good, talented people enriching my life, including my best friend, my boyfriend and all my beloved friends and family, who allow me to just be me, and to share with them all the sinewy observations and curious questions crowding my head—who listen patiently and thoughtfully to me as I fumble around my experiences to get at the heart of what matters, what's really eating away at me and, ultimately, what I will feel compelled to write about. It's so often my friends and family whose feedback and illumination of points help me flesh out an issue. I am also grateful to field experts who take time to talk and hash it out with me; and, to the real, everyday people who share their stories with me in an effort to help others grow. I love you all and I thank you.

About the Author

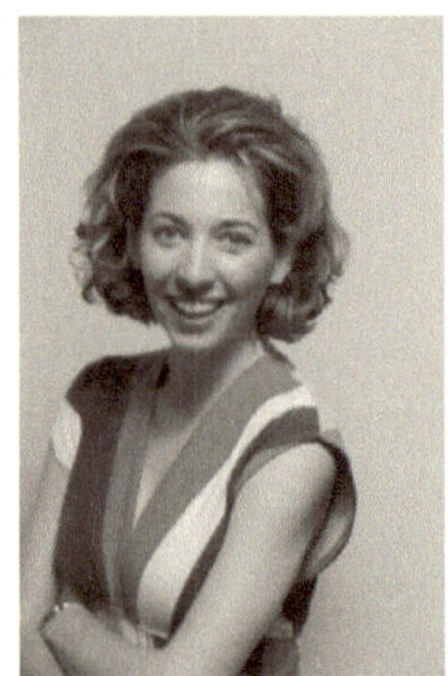

Photo by Jesse Winter

Julie D. Andrews is a writer and editor living in New York City who has been researching, reporting and writing about all aspects of healthy living for nearly 10 years. Her passion is making healthy lifestyle accessible to everyone (those closest to her know the way she ever-so-carefully lets slip the latest juicy tidbits of health research she's read in the form of "Did you know?" advice). Julie is a 2013 Fellow of the Association of Health Care Journalists (AHCJ) and her articles have appeared in print and on the websites of *Prevention, Shape, Men's Fitness, Glamour, Fitness, Cosmo for Latinas, Elle, New York Magazine, LearnVest, iVillage, YourTango, The Huffington Post, TheNest, New York Moves* and more. Connect with her on Twitter @julieDandrews, on Facebook at Julie D. Andrews, and at her website at JulieDAndrews.com.

If you like Julie's work, be among the first to hear about new releases, by sending a request to julie.d.andrews@gmail.com to be added to the **new-release distribution list**.

The digital age has allowed for amazing strides in strengthening the bond between You, the reader, and a writer whose work you are reading. It is a great joy for writers to now be able to see readers' comments about their work online, and the Internet has made these types of connections more possible than ever.

Always remember that a writer works best in solitude, with mere hopes that her words will reach readers like You. Word-of-mouth is key for any new author to succeed in getting her work out into the world, and read. You can play an important role here. If you enjoyed this book, if any part of it spoke to you, if you found yourself relating, nodding your head in agreement or highlighting passages, please consider leaving an online review for *Real Is the New Natural* on Amazon.com. It could make a dramatic difference for this young writer starting down her path, and do much to further the continuation of her writing.

Praise for
Real Is the New Natural

Julie D. Andrews has done a thorough analysis of today's world of health misinformation. How celebrities sell fruit drinks that contain no fruit. How to analyze "natural" and "organic" labels. Reading her book gives you insight on how to unravel a society where it's stars who influence children and adults' eating habits. Her essay on cleansing and dieting, alone, is worth the price of the book, and should be a must-read for everyone. **Ms. Andrews has done her**

research well, and I, as an M.D. author can appreciate her science, and her ability to make reading about it meaningful. *Next time you hear of the latest 'miracle' diet of that movie/rock star, please stop and read 'Real is the New Natural.'"—Murray Grossan, M.D., is an ear, nose, and throat specialist board-certified in head and neck surgery with Cedars-Sinai Medical Center in Los Angeles. Founder of the Grossan Institute, he serves as a consultant to the L.A. County District Attorney, the U.S. Department of Labor, and has authored several books including The Sinus Cure.*

*"Real is the New Natural is a must-read! Andrews cuts through the bs of health marketing, using research to back up the healthiest lifestyle of all: Authentic and balanced living."--**Michelle Herrera Mulligan, Editor in Chief, Cosmopolitan For Latinas***

"A lively, well-researched read. This is such a refreshing take on all the confusing and conflicting health information out there, especially when it comes to nutrition and exercise. ***Julie D. Andrews tells it like it is. This book dispels a lot of harmful misinformation and offers some very useful tips on things like incorporating healthier foods into your life.*** *I'm a much better informed shopper, cook and eater, thanks to this book."—Reader Review on Amazon.com, February 28, 2014*

"Wow, what a fresh look into the crazy world of 'health.' I had a chance to start (and finish) this book while recently stuck in Atlanta traffic due to snow. ***The book really spoke to me and prompted a discussion with my daughter who struggles with image***

insecurities. She is now reading it and we are finally able to talk about this oftentimes sensitive subject. Great book."—*Reader Review on Amazon.com, February 3, 2014*

"Everywhere you look news and media is trending around the healthy lifestyle. It seems like everything I read is how to cook, work out, sleep, or breathe healthy. I'm a career women in my 30s and leading a healthy lifestyle is a priority for my boyfriend and I. Where do we start? I thought I had a good understanding of the falsities that our society has come to accept around celebrity endorsements and weight-sustaining practices, but this book sheds new light on these topics. ***If you're a skeptic or just aren't sure what's right anymore—real, natural, organic? Spend some time with this book, and I promise you—Real Is the New Natural will clear up a lot.***" –*Reader Review on Amazon.com, March 2, 2014*

www.ingramcontent.com/pod-product-compliance
Lightning Source LLC
Chambersburg PA
CBHW050451290526
45786CB00006B/2248

9781497377165